The NET

MW01041354

Study Guide

"a complete reference to successful testtaking"

Contributors

Michael D. Frost, PhD

Mitchell D. Jarvis, BSCS, BSM

Do not give this NET Study Guide away.
This guide will prove helpful throughout your college years.

Publisher: Educational Resources, Inc.
8910 West 62nd Terrace
Shawnee Mission, Kansas 66202

Copyright 2001 (Third Edition) by Educational Resources, Inc. Printed in the United States of America. All rights reserved. No part of the **NET Study Guide** may be reproduced, stored in a retrieval system or transmitted in any form or by any means, electronic, mechanical, photocopying, recording, or otherwise, without the prior written permission of the publisher.

Table of Contents

Introduction

This **NET Study Guide** will help you with *specific* testtaking skills for the Nurse Entrance Test (hereafter referred to as the **NET**), rather than present general ideas and theories of testtaking. We have endeavored to answer your two most urgent questions: What is on the **NET** examination? How can I best prepare for this test?

A recent study reveals that the majority of American colleges and senior high schools do not adequately teach testtaking skills. In this same study, two-thirds of the high school seniors stated that they needed special tutoring prior to all important examinations. Such unfortunate conditions are by no means uncommon. They demonstrate a need for learning specific testtaking skills that help the student achieve all the success possible on the **NET.**

Many poor testtaking behaviors arise from underdeveloped testtaking skills, such as excessive haste, lack of planning, careless reading of questions, and ineffective methods of reading questions. Strict observance of a few simple testtaking guidelines will demonstrate more accurately what you know. These guidelines can improve your understanding of what is required by a test question; therefore, ensuring better scores without "abnormally great effort." For example, numerous investigations have shown that students can often save from one-fourth to one-third of their testtaking time if they systemize their efforts in accordance with well researched, but not well-known, principles of testtaking. We will review with you these principles of testtaking in this **NET Study Guide.**

Effective testtaking approaches will help you understand and remember what you are reading. Most educational handicaps of students are caused by a failure to prepare for a test, correctly. Furthermore, many hours of needless anxiety or confusion might be avoided through knowledge and application of a few practical suggestions. You may be more interested and proficient in studying for a test in one subject, rather than another, but a correct approach to testtaking and study skills will increase your enjoyment and success in all fields of education.

Practice tests, which we have modeled after the **NET**, are provided to give you a good idea of the appearance for each subsection of the test. You can anticipate the test with fewer unknowns and, therefore, less stress and anxiety as you prepare for the **NET.**

Purpose of the NET

Diagnostic Information

The **NET** provides an objective measurement of your *critical reading ability* and compares your ability against the level of mastery required for success in college. Secondly, the **NET** evaluates your level of success with basic mathematics, the math necessary for you to function, not only in your academic courses, but also in your clinical practice following college. Thirdly, the **NET** determines your effective speed in reading college level material. Lastly, the **NET** identifies how you approach study, in general, and identifies which learning approach is most effective for you.

The **NET** strives to academically support you by providing diagnostic information about your basic, academic, processing skills.

The **NET** will not only identify your weaknesses in those processing skills which are necessary for success in college, but the test will enable you to correct your weaknesses prior to entering school. The diagnostic report generated by the **NET** can alert both tutors and the college learning centers to your special needs, so that assistance can be given *before* you experience problems that may tarnish your academic record.

Remember! The **NET** is *not* designed to keep you out of school. It is designed to help you identify which of your academic processing skills must be sharpened before you begin this advanced education.

Use of this NET Study Guide

Follow these steps to effectively profit from this **NET Study Guide**:

Read
Read the entire guide prior to the two practice tests that are provided at the end of the guide.

Pretest
Complete Practice Test A after carefully reading the directions. This is a "mock" test, but accurately follows the format and structure of the **NET**. The reading questions and math problems, although not identical to ones on the **NET**, are written by the same authors who wrote the actual **NET**.

Score
Score Practice Test A using the answer key at the end of the guide.

Chart
Chart your errors for both the reading and mathematics sections of the test.

Study
Study the rationales given for all the reading questions and mathematics problems that you missed. Seek to understand why you missed each test item.

Posttest
Complete Practice Test B. Repeat the steps you completed for scoring/charting Practice Test A.

Final Review
Review the testtaking skills section of this **NET Study Guide**, again, just before taking the **NET** to enhance any testtaking skills in which you may still need help.

Structure of the NET

• ***Reading Comprehension, Basic Math & Learning Styles***

The **NET** will measure both your reading comprehension and math skills and develop an assessment of your learning style.

Your reading comprehension skills will be evaluated at the inferential level of understanding, not the recall level. The math section will begin with addition, subtraction, multiplication and division of whole numbers, then require you to do the same four operations with common fractions, decimals, percentages and basic algebra. The Learning Styles section will ask you to decide whether you agree or disagree with statements.

• ***Multiple Choice Questions***

Each question on both the reading comprehension and math sections of the **NET** will have four answer choices, only one of which is the best answer. The key word here is best. All answers may be true statements, but only one will best fulfill the requirements of the question. No credit will be given for answers that are partially correct.

The Learning Styles assessment will require you to decide whether you agree or disagree with 45 statements. The Learning Styles assessment will be used only for counseling, not as a score by which to admit or keep you from enrolling in a school.

- ***Number of Questions***

The reading comprehension section contains 25 to 35 multiple choice questions. There are 60 math problems and 45 decision statements that seek to determine your learning style.

- ***Time Limits***

You will be given about one minute for each question (30 minutes total) to complete the reading comprehension section and 60 minutes for the math section. You will not be expected to complete the entire reading section of the **NET** before the time is up. You will have 20 minutes to react to the learning styles assessment statements. The entire test will take 110 minutes or a little less than two hours.

- ***Scoring the NET***

Your reading comprehension score will be based upon the number of questions you get correct. Your score will be compared with the scores of many thousands of other examinees who have answered the same questions. The Passing Score will be the low average score established by all those who took the **NET**, nationally.

• ***Reading Comprehension Score***

If your reading comprehension score on the **NET** is below average, you will be given a reading level designation of *Frustration*. This means that even with the benefit of lectures, you would experience more than average difficulty in critically reading college level material.

If your score is within the Average range, you will be given a reading level designation of *Instructional*. This means that with the benefit of lectures, you can be expected to successfully read college level material.

If your score is above the Average range, you will be given a reading level designation of *Independent*. This means that you can successfully read college level material without even the benefit of lectures.

• ***Reading Rate***

A score will be established of your effective reading rate. An average rate of reading is 250 to 400 words per minute. This is the normal "oral" rate at which most people speak. Remember that the normal rate is an average rate. This score will *not* be used as criteria for excluding you from school. However, your diagnostic score could be useful by indicating, to both you and the school, a need for help in order to make it easier for you to read, successfully, the large amount of material assigned in college. Therefore, follow the directions carefully at this part of the **NET** and be truthful. Remember, help cannot be provided by the school if you hide or mask your academic needs.

• ***Mathematics***

The math score is a single score compared against how well thousands of other applicants did on the same 60 questions. If you do well with the basic math operations upon whole numbers, fractions, decimals and percentages, you do not have to get any of the eight algebra questions correct.

• ***Learning Styles***

This section of the **NET** seeks to determine how you best learn and master new information. Which describes you? I am ...

an auditory learner
a visual learner
a social learner
a solitary learner
an oral dependent learner
a writing dependent learner

Again, the Learning Style Assessment will be used only for counseling and has no value or use as admission criteria. Therefore, you should answer the questions carefully and truthfully. The information is diagnostic and will be used in aiding your instructors to teach to your personal learning style(s). Your school wants this information, and this assessment is evidence of a desire by the school program to meet and prepare for your individual needs.

Reading Section of the NET

What is Critical Reading?

The **NET** evaluates your critical reading ability of college level material. Critical reading questions on the **NET** ask you to "read between the lines," that is, to determine the meaning and purpose of what you read. You will be expected to demonstrate that you *understand* a paragraph. The critical reading questions demand more understanding than just identifying vocabulary words, reciting definitions, recalling numbers and literal statements of fact. In college and on the **NET**, you will be expected to state the main idea of a paragraph, its central theme, etc. You will be asked to identify which inferences and conclusions are implied in the paragraphs or groups of paragraphs. You will be asked to predict outcomes based on the paragraph or the entire reading selection.

Paragraph facts and details are taken for granted in college and on the **NET**. It is the summarized meaning and conclusions drawn from the paragraphs that enable you to understand the author's intent and purpose. Once these ideas are understood, you will be able to easily remember details and facts contained in a paragraph.

At first glance, textbooks might look crammed with facts and definitions that must be memorized--and you must memorize these facts and definitions presented in your textbooks. However, this memorization of recall information is made possible and much easier if you have *hooks*, hangers on which to attach and group the new information. These hangers are the main ideas of a paragraph and the central theme uniting paragraphs. The **NET** evaluates how well you can identify these central ideas found within paragraphs and chapter sections.

If your reading skills are weak when you seek to identify and state the central idea of a selection, these skills can be strengthened. You can strengthen your reading skills by completing each practice test in the **NET Study Guide** and then by evaluating the *kinds* of questions you are answering incorrectly.

Therefore, the important value of these practice tests, written by the same authors as the **NET** itself, is to help you carefully determine if there are patterns in your incorrect answers. The answer key for the practice tests not only gives the correct answer, but also the type of critical reading question you missed and the rationale for all answers. Do not berate yourself for missing a question. Strive, instead, to understand the nature of your incorrect answers so that you can improve your critical reading skills.

Remember, all possible answers to the multiple choice question may be correct; however, only one will be the *best* answer, given a careful reading of the question stem.

Critical Reading Summation

A. Reading for the Main Idea

"Main idea" can be defined as a statement of the topic or theme an author has for a paragraph. The author normally states this topic in a sentence near the beginning or end of the paragraph. Your ability to identify the author's intent for a paragraph is necessary if you are to correctly interpret and understand the idea or topic the author has developed. This topic is based on an accurate comprehension of the words, phrases, and the sentences that develop the idea of the paragraph. All the other interpretive reading skills are secondary. If you cannot state the main idea of a paragraph, you will probably not understand the implied meanings of the author in the paragraph, and you may also experience difficulty in summarizing what you have read. Therefore, if you have difficulty stating the general topic of a paragraph, the validity of inferences based upon paragraph facts is weakened. Several inferences can be drawn from facts in a paragraph, but usually only one main idea can be stated for the paragraph. This skill of discovering and stating the main idea of a paragraph can be learned.

B. Inferential Reading

You read inferentially when you draw conclusions from facts and statements within a paragraph. Inferential reading is a process in which you seek to establish a valid, focus statement (a conclusion) from a variety of presenting data. This ability to inferentially read can be learned.

C. Paragraph Function and Significance

Predicting outcomes during reading involves evaluation of validity for inferences that have been made from facts given within the paragraph. Stating the purpose of a paragraph is an example of predicting an outcome from information contained in a paragraph.

Nurses need to learn theoretical and statistical relationships, such as variables which influence high-risk health states. Nurses develop good critical thinking skills in order to process data and daily clinical decisions. Much research related to critical thinking ability has been completed with college students. Critical thinking ability and decision- making skills are closely related cognitive (understanding/thinking) skills. During your college education, you will experience problem-solving processes in which you will collect data utilizing both inductive and deductive reasoning. You will make a hypothesis, which you must be able to support from the detail of your reading or thinking. The **NET** will assess your ability for this critical thinking ability through its critical thinking appraisal.

If you have at least an average intellectual ability, you can learn to be an effective, critical thinker and reader. Since you have graduated from high school or passed your **GED**, you have at ***least*** average or normal intellectual ability. You can succeed in college, but you must seek to sharpen your critical thinking skills so that you can succeed in this career. The **NET** will help you identify those math and reading skill areas of yours which need to be strengthened if you are to demonstrate success, academically.

Remember, the **NET** is *not* used as a tool to exclude you from seeking a career. The **NET** is a diagnostic tool that gives you and the college to which you are applying valuable insight into your preparedness to enter higher education. Given this diagnostic information, you can strengthen your weak academic skills before you enter school. Work carefully with the results of the two practice tests included in this study guide. Learn from your mistakes. Improve your skills. Take the **NET** and demonstrate strong reading and math skills.

Testtaking Strategies for the NET's Reading Comprehension

A. Main Idea

A statement of main idea (1) includes the topic of the paragraph, (2) identifies how this topic ***is*** or ***does*** something, and (3) serves as an umbrella structure for the many details of the paragraph.

The main idea is usually found in a topic sentence found near the beginning of a paragraph. When writing a paragraph, an author normally makes a statement of topic and then proceeds in the paragraph to defend and develop this statement.

Two errors commonly made in identifying the main idea of a paragraph:

Too Narrow. This incorrect statement of main idea looks like an attractive choice because it contains details given in the paragraph. However, this false statement of main idea is narrow in focus and ignores the wider range of details introduced in the paragraph. The details of a paragraph should develop or support the main topic of the paragraph. Therefore, a typical mis-statement of the main idea is said to be *too narrow* in focus to serve as the unifying or main idea of the passage.

Too General. This incorrect statement of the main idea looks attractive because it is broad in scope and obviously references more than just one or two paragraph details. The problem with this statement is that it goes beyond the supporting details presented in the paragraph. For this statement to be a true statement of the main idea, additional information would have to be introduced into the paragraph to support it. Therefore, the problem with this statement of the main idea is the opposite of the topic statement that is *too narrow* in focus. This incorrect statement of the main idea is *too general* in scope and states an aspect of the topic that is beyond the supporting details of the paragraph.

Examples of question stems on the **NET** that ask you to identify a correct statement of main idea for a paragraph:

- Which states the main idea of this paragraph?
- Which is the best statement of main idea for the paragraph?
- Select the main idea for this paragraph.
- The main idea of this paragraph is best revealed by which statement?
- Identify the main idea for this paragraph.

B. Inference

On the **NET**, *inference* refers to a group of words which expresses an unwritten and unstated relationship among the details of a paragraph. An inference, then, expresses an understanding of unstated links between paragraph ideas. This reading process utilizes inductive reasoning.

An inferential question on the **NET** is a conclusion supported by details presented in the paragraph, but not a conclusion that predicts results beyond the unifying idea of the main idea. Inferences that use deductive reasoning, that is, predict results based on the main idea of a paragraph, are separated by the **NET** as another, and higher, processing level of critical reading. Your deductive reasoning and reading ability is evaluated on the **NET** and discussed later in this section of the **NET Study Guide**.

Examples of question stems on the **NET** that require you to identify inferences for a paragraph:

- Identify an inference that can be derived from this paragraph.
- Which is an inference based on the paragraph?
- Which statement is true based upon the paragraph?
- Based on this paragraph, which statement is true?
- Identify a conclusion that can be drawn from this paragraph.
- Which factor in this paragraph supports the topic of soil control?
- Which describes the attitude of the spectators in this paragraph?
- How is sleepwalking characterized in this paragraph?
- Which group experiences the largest number of sleepwalkers, based on paragraphs 31-33?
- What may be assumed by the failure of the neighbors to discover earlier the body of Homer Barron?
- How does Faulkner portray Emily's Negro manservant?

C. Paragraph Function and Significance

Establishing the *theme, purpose* and predicted *outcomes* of a paragraph demonstrates an abstract understanding of a paragraph's function or significance. Stating the theme, purpose and predicted outcome(s) for a paragraph reveals a higher inferential understanding, sometimes involving both inductive and deductive reasoning. Such logical conclusions will not be, concretely, stated in the paragraph or reading selection, as would be a statement of main idea.

Let us look at the terms *theme*, *purpose* and *predicted outcomes*, which require a higher level of critical reading than mere inferential reasoning does with details or ideas *within* a paragraph.

Theme

Typically, a statement of *theme* is only a phrase, not a sentence. A statement of theme would resemble a short book title, which is usually a symbolically stated topic of the story. The significance of the title is only completely understood when the entire book has been read. Some examples:

To Kill a Mockingbird
Little Women
Red Storm Rising
Hunt for Red October
Pride and Prejudice
War and Peace

Question stems on the **NET** that would ask you to identify the theme of a paragraph or selection will look like the following:

- Which would be a statement of theme for this paragraph?
- Identify the central, unifying theme of the last 3 paragraphs.
- What is the common theme of this article?

Purpose

The *purpose* of a paragraph goes beyond a statement of either main idea or topic. Stating the purpose of a selection is to make a value judgment about "why" a selection was written.

Question stems on the NET that would ask you to identify the *purpose* of a paragraph or selection will look like the following:

- Identify the purpose of paragraphs J-L.
- Which is the purpose of paragraph M?
- Which is the best statement of purpose for paragraph Q?
- Which is a statement of purpose that can be supported by paragraphs B-F?

Predicting Outcomes

To *predict an outcome* from a paragraph is to project an action, a result, that is based upon the premise developed by the paragraph, as supported by the details or reasoning evolved within a paragraph. A predicted outcome of a paragraph is the result of inductive reasoning supported by the main idea and based on possible inferences from the details and facts within a paragraph or larger, written work.

Question stems on the **NET** will ask you to predict an outcome, identify a result based on the ideas developed in one or several paragraphs. These stems will look like the following:

- As discussed in paragraph J, which behavior during noctambulation seems to be directly related to dream content and symbolic expression?
- Which would be an outcome from paragraph F?
- An outcome resulting from paragraph G.
- Which is a true statement based on these two paragraphs?
- Based on these two paragraphs, which is a true conclusion?

35 General Testtaking Strategies for the NET

Be calm as you prepare to take the **NET**. In particular, utilize the following testtaking hints to better demonstrate your true critical reading ability with the paragraphs that make up the reading part of the test.

1. Read and follow all directions carefully.

2. Glance at the type of questions that make up the section of the test you are assigned. Note the format or structure of each question. Note that the questions are multiple choice and have four answer options. On the **NET**, the questions do not start easy and become difficult. There will be no recall questions that simply expect you to remember just the literal facts of a paragraph. Every attempt has been made to write questions that require you to "read between the lines" and cause you to demonstrate a higher than average recall level of understanding. Therefore, begin with the first question and work your way through the reading selections, answering each question as it is presented.

3. Carefully use the two practice tests in this **NET Study Guide**. Then, there will be no surprises for you when you

sit down to take the **NET**. The "look" of the test will be familiar, as well as the type and difficulty level of both the reading questions and math problems.

4. Relax and treat the **NET** as if it were *another practice test*, except that you will have a time limit in which you must work.

5. Before you read a paragraph, first look at the questions presented for the individual paragraph. *Read the question stem part of each question* to get a "purpose for reading" in mind, before you read the paragraph. Do not take time to read all the A, B, C, D options. However, reading the question stem gives you a purpose for reading: for a definition, a numerical amount, a main idea, an inference, etc. Any time that you read a paragraph or selection with a question in mind, your reading comprehension will be improved, as well as your answering time because you have established a focus for your reading. You will also find that you can concentrate with less effort, and, of course, this leads to increased understanding of the paragraph.

6. Reject the temptation to select an answer that appears to be a true statement until you have *read all options.* Although an answer might be a true statement, a later option may be a better answer. The best answer is the desired one, even though others may be true or partially true statements.

7. Above all, *guard against feelings of resentment* or *anger* toward the test proctor due to any frustration or anxiety you may experience during the test. The test proctor will help you do your best by keeping noise to a minimum, seeing that the temperature and lighting are right, supplying you with extra pencils, answering those questions that can be answered about the test, etc.

8. *Relax.* Keep calm, especially before the examination. Some tension is natural and serves to keep you mentally and physically alert, but too much tension may bring about mental blocking. Blocking usually leads to frustration, worry, and more tension which, in turn, may bring on more blocking, thus compounding the difficulty.

9. One way to avoid accumulating excess tension is to *anticipate your needs*. Do not be in a rush. Allow plenty of time to accomplish all the things you have to do before the test. Such activities might be attending to toilet needs, comfort in clothing, etc.

10. Once in the examination room, you can *keep tension under control* by concentrating on some points you wish to remember. Once the examination begins, exclude thoughts of failure from your mind by focusing on the examination itself.

11. Do not go into the testing room with a *negative attitude*, such as, "I'm sure I won't pass," or even a neutral attitude, such as, "Let the chips fall where they may."

12. To do your best, you must *think positively*. On the other hand, an *overconfident* attitude may keep you from being as alert as you might be.

13. Do not believe that the only questions you are capable of answering correctly are those you know right away. By working hard, you can often raise your score considerably. Through persistence and the use of principles discussed in this **NET Study Guide**, you can overcome the tendency to underachieve on the **NET**.

14. Remember, always work hard throughout the *full time allowed*. Do not come into the examination room with thoughts of leaving early or doing anything less than your best. Stick to the job!

15. CONCENTRATE. *Avoid distractions.* Once in the examination room, do not be distracted by the actions of others. This can interfere with your success on the material presented to you. Before the **NET** begins, preoccupy yourself by going over in your mind the testtaking skills you have practiced as preparation. Then when the exam begins, think only about the examination. To eliminate other potential sources of distraction during an examination, avoid sitting near a window, if you can help it, or beside your significant other.

16. *Use time wisely.* Do not spend excessive time on any one question. It is urgent that time be budgeted to permit an honest attempt at every question. Never spend more than one minute per question or problem. You must have time to attempt all questions/problems.

17. *Read directions and questions carefully.* Remember what the time limits are, how to answer the questions, and how they will be scored. Be especially alert to the key items, knowing that just one word misread or misinterpreted may lead to an incorrect answer.

18. *Attempt every question.* Remember that questions which look complicated and involved may not be so difficult once you get into them. Each question is worth one point, the same point as every other question. So answer every question, even if it is just your best guess.

19. Choose the answer which *the test maker intended.* You hurt no one but yourself when you read into a question qualifications and interpretations clearly not intended by the test maker. For example,

> *Thomas Jefferson wrote the Declaration of Independence. (True or False)*

Some students might object to answering *true*, saying that four other men were also on the writing committee. The sophisticated testtaker, however, would answer *true* because he would realize that this was the answer which the test maker intended for the particular level and purpose for the test.

Now, if the test maker had intended to find out whether you were aware that the document was written by a committee, the test item might read like this:

> *Thomas Jefferson, alone, wrote the Declaration of Independence. (True or False)*

On standardized tests, such as the **NET**, always choose the option which you believe has the greatest chance of being correct, even though others have merit and even though the chosen option is not completely satisfactory.

20. *Anticipate the answer*, then look for it. Always anticipate what the answer will be like. Then look for it among the options. This step should be accomplished very quickly. Though you may not anticipate exactly the answer that is called for, you can often anticipate some of the logical characteristics of the correct answer. For example,

> *Why is Cavalieri's Principle important in solid geometry?*

Assuming that you may not know the answer, you could still logically anticipate that the correct answer will clearly be a *reason* why the principle is *important*. On that basis, options which are not reasons, or reasons which are not important, may be eliminated, freeing you to center your attention on the remaining option(s). Let us now apply this principle of anticipation to a critical thinking question.

Why is Cavalieri's Principle important in solid geometry?

a) *It shows that the surface area of a cube of side "s" is* $6s^2$
b) *It contradicts the principles of Euclid and Gauss*
c) *It provides the basis for finding the volume formulae for many solids*

This question is especially difficult if you have never heard of Cavalieri's Principle. Nevertheless, by using the principle of anticipation, you can object to option (a) because it seemed too specific to have an important bearing on the wide field of solid geometry. Option (b) should also seem unattractive because it is negative in its "contribution" to solid geometry and because it is implausible. Option (c) possesses the anticipated ingredients of being a reason and having both a wide and an important bearing on the field of solid geometry.

21. *Consider all the alternatives.* Read and consider all the options, even though the first option may have all the characteristics which you anticipated. This procedure of suspended judgment is especially pertinent when dealing with multiple-choice tests, such as the **NET**, which is a "pick-the-best-answer" variety. In such a test, all the options to a question may be true, but one is the best. Because many students do jump at the first plausible option, test makers frequently place their most attractive "decoy" first.

22. *Relate options to the question.* When the anticipated answer is not among the options, promptly discard it and concentrate on the given options by systematically considering how well each one answers the question. If you continue to hold on to your answer (which you may think is quite ingenious) or if you consider the options without

continually relating them to the original question, then these pitfalls await you.

> **First**, by not relinquishing the anticipated answer, you increase the tendency to choose an option which bears only a superficial resemblance to it. You can still be saved from this pitfall by asking yourself whether this "close cousin" is the correct answer to this specific question. This procedure forces you to relate options to questions.
>
> **Second**, when none of the options listed appeals to you, you may be tempted to alter one or more words in an option to make it "correct." Do not force the answer; rather, test each real option against the real questions.
>
> **Third**, if you ponder the options without relating them continually to the question, you may pick an option which is correct in itself, but incorrect as it relates to the question. It is possible that all the listed options are correct statements, but only one of them will be the correct answer to the question.

For example,

> *A spinning baseball curves because:*
>
> *a) the airspeeds on either side of the ball are unequal*
> *b) the ball is spherical*
> *c) the momentum of the ball is equal to the product of its mass and velocity*

Since both options (b) and (c) are true, many students would narrow their attention to these, probably choosing (c) because the words momentum, mass, and velocity pertain to a thrown baseball. Such narrowing of attention is akin to "tunnel vision". To avoid this pitfall, remember never to deal with options in isolation. (a) is the correct answer.

23. Just as *correct* statements can be wrong answers to some questions, so can wrong statements be correct answers to other questions. "The world is flat" is an *incorrect* statement, but it is the correct answer to the following question:

> *"In the 15th century most European mariners feared to sail westward on the Atlantic because they believed that . . ."*

This illustrates, again, the need to relate the options to the question.

24. *Balance options* against each other. When several options look good, or even if none look good, compare them with each other. If two options are highly similar, study them to find what makes them different. For example,

> *The French Revolution of the 18th century was mainly the result of which?*
>
> *a) American objections to the extension of slavery*
> *b) the oppression by the Parisian middle classes of the French nobility*
> *c) the oppression by the Bourbon monarchs of the French peasantry*
> *d) overproduction of food*

Most students would probably eliminate options (a) and (d) as unlikely answers, leaving both (b) and (c) for further consideration. Options (b) and (c) are similar in that they both deal with the topic of *oppression.* But they are different in that (b) asserts that the nobility was oppressed by the people, a most unlikely situation; and (c) points out that the nobility oppressed the people, a most usual and likely situation. Option (c) is correct, of course.

25. Use *logical reasoning.* Actively reason through the questions. Some students passively stare at math or reading problems, hoping that correct answers will somehow pop up as if by magic. This is wishful thinking. Correct solutions come about when thinking about each part of the problem as aggressive and continual.

To free you to concentrate on fewer options, eliminate those which you know are incorrect, as well as those which obviously do not fit the "promise" or requirements of the question. For example,

The nose:

a) develops during gastrulation
b) has two movable joints
c) is structured in part by the turbinals
d) is an organ of balance

The sophisticated testtaker would eliminate options (b) and (d) and choose between (a) and (c).

Logical reasoning is exemplified in a situation in which, say, you recognize that two or more options are correct, and that one of the remaining options encompasses both of these. In such a situation, always choose the more encompassing option. The following example and explanation will help to make this principle clear.

Which of the following cities is in the state of New York?

a) Syracuse
b) Rome
c) Albany
d) All of the above

The test-wise student who knew that two of the cities (*Syracuse* and *Albany*) were in New York but who had never heard of *Rome*, New York, would automatically choose the encompassing answer (d) *All of the above*.

26. Look for *specific determiners*. Some specific determiners are such words as *rarely* and *usually* which qualify the main statement of a question. Many students find these qualifying words perplexing. We cannot guarantee that you will never find them perplexing, but we do have some advice based on experience.

Since so many statements have exceptions, true statements often contain qualifying words and false ones often do not. But you cannot rely totally on this technique, because an experienced test writer carefully mixes up the items so that some statements with qualifiers are false and some statements without qualifiers are correct. Another class of specific determiners is exact terms such as *always* and *none*. These words should be taken literally. When a statement is qualified by the word *always*, it means not 98 or 99 percent of the time, but a full 100 percent of the time.

Some other *absolute* determiners:

Always	All
Never	None

27. Watch for *qualifying* words:

More	Most
Least	Best
First	Better

These words should be flag wavers for you. An answer might be correct, but if after carefully reading the question, is it the *best* answer? All the answers may be partially correct, but only one truly fits the requirements of the question as the best statement of main idea, the best statement of an inference drawn from the reading passage, or the best statement of a predictable outcome from the passage.

Remember: All answer options may be correct, but only one option may be the **best, least, most,** etc. correct than the others. This one option, and only one, will then be the one you should select.

28. Look for combination *umbrella* and *priority* choices. An example would be the following question:

> *Which chair is best for a client to use the first time out of bed after back surgery?*
>
> *A. Soft chair with a low seat*
> *B. Rocking chair*
> *C. Straight chair with a high back*
> *D. An armchair with a firm, secure cushion*

Key testtaking words in the question stem are **first** and **back** surgery.

Common sense would suggest that choices "A" and "B" would provide little support for the back surgery client, and, therefore, both choices would probably be incorrect ones. Choice "C" offers support for the back. Option "D", however, would be the best choice because what is desirable in option "C" is contained in option "D," plus the additional support of the chair's arms.

29. Watch for *negative words* and *prefixes*: contraindicated, not, un-, in-, and im-, etc. These words and prefixes change the focus of a test item. Instead of searching among the possible answers for a positive answer, you are required to focus on a negative option. The question, then, has become

a kind of true/false one. You may be asked to decide what you would not do, or what would not be an expected outcome. Be aware of this change in focus from "what would happen" to "what would not." Good test writers try to avoid the negative question stem, but sometimes they appear.

30. Avoid choosing the *"different"* answer. Do not choose an answer just because it appears different than the others. For instance, one answer might be a verb and the other three options might be adverbs. Just because one is a different part of speech is not a reason for choosing it. Normally, test writers feel that their correct answers "stand out" as it is, and the last thing they would do is leave it looking odd. The correct option will usually blend with the others.

31. Do not look for a pattern of answers on your answer sheet. If the last four questions have had answers in the B position, for instance, do not expect the next answer also to be B. A good test writer will rotate the correct answers through the A, B, C and D positions so that this will not happen. The goal of a good test writer is to have the correct answer equally placed in all four positions.

32. Answers are usually of average length. The correct answer is usually of average length. Again, the test writer is seeking to keep the correct answer from standing out among the incorrect ones.

33. Look for determiner words used in a question which denote *sequence* priority. Some obvious words could be *first, last, initial, immediate, etc.* A question might ask you to decide what is the *first* action required by a paragraph or reading selection, or it might ask you what is the last point the paragraph developed.

The following are taken from question stems. Italics have been added for your benefit. Question writers will not usually be this helpful:

> What is the *priority* assessment you would make *at this time*?
>
> What is the *priority* assessment to be made immediately *after* the mother gives birth?
>
> What is the *first* thing you would do for this client?
>
> Which is the *last* step of this procedure?

34. Look for priority words where value is the important focus of the determiner word, not sequence. The following is an example of a question containing such a priority word:

> *During the <u>initial</u> infertility interview, what is your <u>primary</u> objective?*

What is important to you in the above is that all the answers may be real objectives of the person providing care. However, you are asked to evaluate the objectives and determine which is the primary or important one. Look for key words in questions that ask for you to assess *value*.

35. Finally, it is possible to read a paragraph on the test several times and still get very little out of it. On the other hand, if you read it only once or twice, but in the right way, you will get a great deal out of it. In the latter case, chances are that you followed certain practical rules of testtaking.

That is, first read the appropriate questions directed at specific paragraph(s) to get a focus for your reading and then read the paragraph(s). In this way you determined the test writer's purpose for the reading:

1. *determination of the main idea or central theme*
2. *deciding whether a statement is true based upon the paragraph(s)*
3. *you need to criticize, compare, digest, ask questions and/or discover answers*
4. *or you are to apply some of the other procedures of efficient learning*

It is, in fact, easier to approach a test in the correct way, than it is to use wasteful or incorrect methods.

Summary of General Testtaking Strategies

Self-Analysis

Anyone who wishes to do so can improve testtaking skills. It is necessary, however, to discover your own most urgent testtaking problems. Of course, the conscientious application of attention and energy is indispensable. With such application, learning how to take tests should make your testtaking efforts more direct, effective, and successful. But you must analyze your own needs and select the hints that will be of greatest assistance in your situation.

Are you reading the selections too quickly, without good understanding and retention?

Is your focus on the test requirements well balanced and comprehensive?

Background for Comprehension

The process of learning may be compared to the construction of a house on a sound foundation; every useful idea you can relate to the new material will form an added basis for clear understanding of what you have read.

Careful Reading

Resist the temptation to be satisfied with quick reading and casual reflection. You may feel that you have understood an author's principal ideas, so that reflection does not seem attractive or worthwhile, but remember that superficial reading will seldom ensure thorough understanding or later recall of its important points. Therefore, you should take time to read the question, then think seriously about each of the options. True, there are times during the test when you may wish only to skim the question or the paragraphs, but never mistake skimming for reflective reading. For the latter, careful rereading is necessary, together with comparisons and contrasts, critical reactions and the analyses of implications.

> *Reject the temptation to guess the answer unless you have an honest basis for believing it to be probably correct.*

> *Whenever you can do so quickly, associate questions with each other and with as many important ideas as you can develop.*

Reading Rate Section of the NET

Definitions

The **NET** will produce one of three scores for your reading rate, and these are defined below.

Frustration Rate
If you generate a Frustration Rate score, it is estimated that your reading rate is so slow that you will be unable to complete all the reading required of you in college, given all of the other daily time requirements generally demanded of students. This rate can be dramatically improved with work. A Frustration Rate score will not effect whether or not you are admitted to a school. It will simply indicate an area in which you must work effectively to read and understand your textbooks in which you will receive reading assignments.

Instructional Rate
If your score on the **NET** generates this rating, you would be reading at a rate of 250 to 400 words per minute with at least 70% comprehension. This is the normal college rate of reading and is expected of most college students.

Independent Rate
If your score on the **NET** generates this reading rate, the **NET** is estimating that you read in excess of 450 words per minute with at least 70% comprehension. This would be an excellent accomplishment, but not a necessary one for a college student.

Strategies for Increasing Your Speed of Reading

As a rule, outstanding students are fast readers. They cover written material rapidly, gaining time for rereading and reviewing. The **NET** measures your reading rate for textbook material during the reading comprehension section.

The average person reads all printed material at the same rate, which is an oral reading rate of 250 to 450 words per minute with a comprehension level of 70%.

Some readers read too slowly because of certain correctable bad habits and unfavorable environmental conditions. Think back to your past experiences and decide whether some of the following common causes of excessively slow reading apply to you.

1. *Failure to keep in mind a definite purpose for reading.* If you allow your attention to wander instead of concentrating on the important purposes for your reading, you will be apt to waste time on trivial points and reduce your rate considerably. Therefore, analyze the results you wish to get from your reading (information, main ideas, topic themes, inferences, etc.) and check them off mentally as soon as you achieve them. This technique prevents wasting too much time on nonessentials. It will help you to increase your rate of reading most types of subject matter with adequate understanding.

2. *Excessive attention to single words.* Sometimes it is necessary to stop and analyze complex technical words to ascertain the test writer's intended meaning. But it is a common mistake to overdo this type of word analysis to such an extent that the attention wanders far afield from

the question requirements. Analyze significant terms which contribute to the meaning, but concentrate on the main ideas, without ignoring apparently minor words, such as not, or and the like, which can change the importance of an entire passage.

3. *Flexibility or lack of same.* The ability to read at high speed may be necessary in reading for information, but it is generally of little importance in reading material that requires hard thinking and analysis, such as the reading comprehension section of the **NET**. A slow pace is essential when you are reading for difficult purposes. Nevertheless, do a quick preview of the test question, then skim rapidly through the appropriate paragraph(s). Use good judgment in adapting your rate to the kind of context you are reading.

This type of subject matter presented in the **NET** requires you to carefully read difficult passages, evaluate purposes and inferences, as well as central themes and main ideas. A preliminary quick reading of the question must be followed by careful, thoughtful reading. Therefore, develop the approach of reading the text after you have established a purpose for reading, ***determined, first, by your reading of the test questions.***

If your rate of reading score is far below average, you should begin remedial steps, including extensive practice in reading with the deliberate objective of increasing your rate.

Both speed and comprehension are inseparable factors of effective reading and cannot be measured independently of each other. Fast reading of text is useless unless you gain a clear understanding of what you have read. Very slow reading, however, gives no assurance of adequate comprehension, especially if it obscures the over-all view of the reading selection or interrupts the smooth flow of ideas. Your objective on the **NET** should be to read slow enough to understand what you read, but to maintain a reading rate fast enough to cover the reading selection within the available time. The most satisfactory rate will vary with the nature of the text, *your purpose in reading*, and your skill in reading with comprehension. Due to these factors, some readers can be expected to read more rapidly than others, but most readers can reach a high level of efficiency if they will take the trouble to analyze their own habits and needs and then apply remedial measures.

• *Methods of Increasing Speed*
As a rule, outstanding students are fast readers. They cover ground rapidly, gaining time for rereading and reviewing.

• *Self-Analysis*
Some readers read too slowly because of certain correctable bad habits and unfavorable environmental conditions. Think back to your past experience and decide whether or not some of these common causes of excessively slow reading apply in your case.

• *Flexibility*
The ability to read at high speed may be necessary in reading for information, but it is generally of little importance in reading material requiring hard thinking and analysis. A slow pace is essential when you are studying a difficult text. Nevertheless, a quick preview of a reading selection, skimming rapidly through it, can be quite useful before you begin slow reading of the material. Use good judgment in adapting your rate to the kind of book you are reading. It would be unwise to dash through one of Shakespeare's plays once or twice and assume adequate understanding. This type of subject matter requires you to review difficult passages and scenes, ask questions about

the events and dialogue, analyze the language, style, and structure, and identify yourself with the characters as if they were living persons whom you could observe in life situations. A preliminary quick reading of such material must be followed by slow, careful rereading. On the other hand, if you are consulting a reference work to find specific information, you can read at a high rate without detailed analysis. Therefore, develop the ability to read at high speed, but use the ability wisely, to ensure the degree of mastery you wish to achieve.

Mathematics Section of the NET

I. Fractions

As time went on, man (and woman) needed a way of indicating or expressing *parts* of whole things, such as half of a bushel of wheat, three out of four pieces of one pie, etc. So *two* new number systems were developed to express these quantities. The first number system to express *parts* was called the common fraction number system. The second kind of number system to express *parts* of things was named the decimal fraction system, commonly just called the decimal system.

You were taught to add, subtract, multiply and divide common and decimal fractions by the end of fourth grade. This was a lot of math for an 9-year-old to master, but most students get through it with at least a general understanding. However, your elementary teachers continued to review these two number systems and the four calculations with them for the next four years.

Generally, by the end of first year algebra, you had been taught how to add, subtract, multiply and divide a number system called *integers*. This was the number system of positive and negative numbers. You were not only taught to add and subtract in this new number system, but you were also taught how to multiply and divide integers. You were taught to solve for first one unknown, commonly expressed as x, and then to solve for two unknowns. You were then taught to solve both linear and quadric equations, and this involved addition, subtraction, multiplication and division processes. By the way, the rules for multiplying and dividing fractions in algebra are the same rules as those you learned in the fourth grade for common fractions.

In fact, something to keep in mind as you review math is that your training in mathematics has been very sequential, and for a very good reason. Math is very sequential. You can not succeed with multiplication and division calculations, if you cannot both add and subtract. The mastery of each number system (whole numbers, common fractions, decimal fractions, percentages, algebra, etc.) is dependent on how well you mastered the proceeding number system. You cannot be successful with operations of decimals if you cannot do the same operations (add, subtract, etc.) with common fractions.

We will assume that you have mastered the four calculations with whole numbers. If you have not, get a friend or a tutor to drill you on the multiplication tables, and division facts.

We would like to start your review of mathematics with the number system introduced to you in the fourth grade, the common fraction system. The common fraction system can express parts of a "whole" thing as $\frac{1}{2}$, $\frac{3}{4}$, $\frac{5}{8}$, etc. The bottom part of the common fraction expression is named the *denominator* and indicates how many parts a whole thing is divided into. The top part of the common fraction is called the *numerator*, and indicates how many of these parts are being counted. Therefore, $\frac{1}{2}$ says that the original thing (a cake, a pie, a bushel of wheat, etc., is divided into two parts, and just one (1) of these original pieces is being counted.

> Now, your elementary and high school math teachers might want to talk about the *size* of the parts, but for the sake of simplifying our discussion, we are going to talk about the *number* of parts of a whole thing. After all, your elementary and high school teachers have had their chance with you. Now it is our turn to explain fractions; that is, if you feel the review will be helpful. We guarantee that a review of math will help you on the **NET**, if it has been a few years since you computed common and

decimal fractions, or completed first year algebra. Back to the discussion of common fractions.

An expression stated as $\frac{3}{4}$ says that the whole thing, whatever that is, is divided into four parts and you are working with three of those four parts.

Many medication preparations are prescribed and prepared in fractions. You will need to know how to calculate medication dosages when fractions are used. A fraction is a portion or piece of a whole that indicates division of that whole into equal units or parts. For example, if you divide an apple into four equal parts, each part is considered to be $\frac{1}{4}$ of the apple. Each section is a fraction of the apple. Fractions are made up of a numerator and a denominator. The top number of the fraction is the numerator and the bottom number is the denominator. Look at the example below:

$\frac{2}{3}$ - where 2 is the numerator and 3 is the denominator

Remember the following rule:

☞ ***The Numerator is the Number on the Top of the Fraction and the Denominator is the Number on the Bottom of the Fraction.***

A. The Denominator of a Fraction

The denominator of a fraction tells you the number of equal parts into which the whole has been divided. For example, if you divide something into 4 equal parts, each part would be expressed as a fraction that has the denominator of 4. That is, each part would be equal to $\frac{1}{4}$. If you divide something into eight equal parts, the denominator is 8, and each part would be equal to $\frac{1}{8}$.

If you sliced two pizzas, one into 8 slices and the other into 4 slices, you will notice that the pizza that is divided into $\frac{1}{8}$'s has smaller portions than the pizza that is divided into $\frac{1}{4}$'s. The reason is that the fraction $\frac{1}{8}$ is less than $\frac{1}{4}$. Even though $\frac{1}{8}$ has a larger denominator (8) than $\frac{1}{4}$ (4), it is a smaller fraction. This is an important concept to understand: that is, the bigger the number in the denominator, the smaller the fraction or pieces of the whole. To clarify, consider these examples:

$\frac{1}{2}$ is greater than $\frac{1}{4}$

$\frac{1}{8}$ is greater than $\frac{1}{16}$

$\frac{1}{9}$ is greater than $\frac{1}{10}$

Remember the following rule:

☞ ***The Bigger the Number in the Denominator, the Smaller the Pieces (or Fractions) of the Whole.***

B. The Numerator of a Fraction

The numerator tells you how many of the equal parts you have. For example, the numerator 3 in the fraction $\frac{3}{4}$ tells you that you have three equal parts that are each worth $\frac{1}{4}$.

The numerator 2 in the fraction $\frac{2}{5}$ tells you that you have 2 equal parts that are each worth $\frac{1}{5}$.

C. Fractions that are Equal To, More Than, or Less Than One

The rules below tell you how to decide if a fraction is equal to one (a whole thing), more than one, or less than one.

☞ ***If the Numerator and Denominator Are Equal to Each Other, the Fraction Is Equal to One.***

EXAMPLES: $\frac{5}{5} = 1$, $\frac{10}{10} = 1$

☞ ***If the Numerator is Greater Than the Denominator, the Fraction Is Equal to or More Than One.***

EXAMPLES: $\frac{3}{2} > 1$, $\frac{5}{4} > 1$, $\frac{8}{3} > 1$

☞ ***If the Numerator is Less Than the Denominator, the Fraction Is Equal to Less Than One. (The Symbol < means Less Than One or points to the smaller quantity.)***

EXAMPLES: $\frac{1}{3} < 1$, $\frac{2}{5} < 1$, $\frac{1}{20} < 1$

D. Mixed Numbers and Improper Fractions

Fractions that are equal to more than one may be written in two ways: as mixed numbers or as improper fractions. Mixed Numbers consist of a whole number and a fraction written together.

EXAMPLES: $2\frac{1}{2}$, $3\frac{2}{3}$, $4\frac{4}{5}$

Improper Fractions are fractions that have a numerator greater than the denominator. Mixed numbers can be changed to improper fractions. For example, $1\frac{1}{2}$ can be changed to $\frac{3}{2}$. The following routine tells you how to change a mixed number to an improper fraction.

• ***Changing a Mixed Number to an Improper Fraction***

To change a mixed number to an improper fraction follow these steps:

1. Multiply the denominator of the fraction by the whole number. That is, if you have the fraction of $2\frac{3}{5}$, you would multiply 2 x 5, which equals 10.

2. Then, add the numerator of the fraction (3) to the answer you got when you multiplied the denominator by the whole number in the above step (10). With the example above, this means that you would add 3 to 10, and get the answer of 13.

3. The answer that you got in the above step (13) becomes the new numerator of the new single fraction. The denominator in the original mixed fraction (which is 5 in this example) stays the same, because the whole things were each divided into 5 pieces.

4. The mixed number $2\frac{3}{5}$ becomes the improper fraction $\frac{13}{5}$.

Improper fractions can also be changed to mixed numbers. For example, the fraction $\frac{5}{3}$ can be changed to $1\frac{2}{3}$. Often, when you are working the mathematics for a given problem, you will need to work with improper fractions. However, if you get a final answer that is an improper fraction, convert it to a mixed number. For example, it is better to say "I have $1\frac{2}{3}$ apples " than to say "I have $\frac{5}{3}$ apples." Look at the rule below which tells you how to change an improper fraction to a mixed number.

- ***Changing an Improper Fraction to a Mixed Number***

To change an improper fraction to a mixed number, follow these steps:

1. Divide the top number (numerator) by the bottom number (denominator). If you use the example of $\frac{7}{3}$, this means you would divide 7 by 3:

$$
\begin{array}{r}
2 \\
3\overline{)7} \\
-\underline{\;6} \\
1
\end{array}
$$

2. The number that you get when you divide the numerator by the denominator becomes the whole number of the mixed number. In the above example, (2) becomes the whole number.

3. The number that you have left over (1 in the example above) becomes the numerator of the fraction that goes with the whole number to make it a mixed number. Using the above example, your answer would look like this so far: $2\frac{1}{?}$.

4. The original denominator of the fraction of the mixed number (which is 3 in this case) becomes the denominator of the fraction of Equivalent or Equal Fractions

5. The result of this process produces: $2\frac{1}{3}$.

- ***Changing Fractions with Different Denominators to Equivalent or Equal Fractions***

When you are working problems with fractions, it is sometimes necessary to change a fraction to a more understandable but equivalent fraction. For example, it is better to express $\frac{3}{6}$ as $\frac{1}{2}$ or $\frac{2}{6}$ as $\frac{1}{3}$. You can make a new fraction that has the same value by either multiplying or dividing both the numerator and the denominator by the same number.

$\frac{3}{4}$ can be changed to $\frac{6}{8}$ by multiplying both the numerator and the denominator by 2.

$$\frac{3 \times 2}{4 \times 2} = \frac{6}{8}$$

$\frac{6}{9}$ can be changed to $\frac{2}{3}$ by dividing both the numerator and the denominator by 3.

$$\frac{6 \div 3}{9 \div 3} = \frac{2}{3}$$

It is important to remember that you can change the numerator and the denominator of a fraction and still keep the same value so long as you follow the following rule:

☞ ***When Changing a Fraction, You Must Do the Same Thing (Multiply or Divide by the Same Number) to the Numerator and to the Denominator in Order to Keep the Same Value.***

To determine that both fractions have equal value, multiply the opposite numerators and denominators. For example, if $\frac{2}{3} = \frac{4}{6}$, then the product of 2 x 6 will equal the product of 3x4.

$$2 \times 6 = 12 \text{ and } 3 \times 4 = 12$$

E. Simplifying, or Reducing Fractions

It is often easier to work with fractions that have been simplified, or reduced to the lowest terms. This means that the numerator and the denominator are the smallest numbers that can still represent the fraction or piece of the whole. For example, $\frac{4}{10}$ can be reduced to $\frac{2}{5}$; $\frac{4}{8}$ can be reduced to $\frac{1}{2}$. It is important to know how to reduce (or simplify) a fraction. The following rule outlines the steps for reducing a fraction to the lowest terms:

• ***To Reduce a Fraction to its Lowest Terms***

1. Study both the numerator and denominator and determine the *largest number* that can go evenly into both the numerator and the denominator. For example suppose you are asked to reduce the fraction $\frac{8}{16}$. The largest number that will go into both the numerator (8) and the denominator (16) is 8.

2. Divide both the numerator and the denominator by the number that you determined will go evenly into both of them. Using the example above, this means you would do the following:

$$\frac{8 \div 8}{16 \div 8} = \frac{1}{2}$$

Now stop and think. If you have 8 out of the 16 parts into which you divided something, you have $\frac{1}{2}$ of it. We are still expressing the same amount, but just in a different fashion.

F. Addition of Fractions

Fractions can be added whether the denominators are like (same) or unlike.

Steps to add Fractions with Like Denominators

1. Add the numerators. For example, to add $\frac{2}{7} + \frac{3}{7}$, add the numerators 2 + 3 = 5.

2. Place the new numerator over the like denominator that remains the same.

3. Reduce to lowest terms, if necessary.

4. Change any improper fraction to a mixed number.

Steps to add Fractions with Unlike Denominators

1. Find a common denominator. The easiest way to find a common denominator is to multiply all the denominators of the expression. For example, to add $\frac{1}{3}+\frac{2}{5}$ find a common denominator by multiplying both of the denominators 3 x 5 which equals 15.

2. Change the unlike fractions to like fractions, by dividing the common denominator of 15 by the denominator of each fraction.

$$15 \div 3 = 5 \text{ and } 15 \div 5 = 3.$$

3. Take each new quotient and multiply it by the numerator of each fraction. Thus,

$$\frac{1 \times 5}{3 \times 5} = \frac{5}{15} \text{ and } \frac{2 \times 3}{5 \times 3} = \frac{6}{15}$$

4. Add the fraction and reduce if necessary.

$$\frac{5}{15} + \frac{6}{15} = \frac{11}{15}$$

G. Subtraction of Fractions

Fractions can be subtracted whose denominators are the same or unlike.

- ***Subtraction of Fractions with Like Denominators***

1. To subtract fractions with like denominators simply subtract the numerators. If you need to subtract $\frac{3}{8}$ from $\frac{7}{8}$, simply subtract 3 from 7, which equals 4.
2. Place the new numerator over the like denominator that remains the same. Place the new numerator 4 over 8.
3. Reduce to lowest terms, if necessary. Reduce $\frac{4}{8}$ to $\frac{1}{2}$.

$$\frac{7}{8} - \frac{3}{8} = \frac{4}{8} \; or \; \frac{1}{2}$$

- ***Subtraction of Fractions with Unlike Denominators***

You will probably never need to subtract unlike fractions or fractions with a mixed number to calculate dosage problems. However, both will be presented here briefly in case you want to review the steps.

1. Find a common denominator. To subtract $\frac{3}{5}$ from $\frac{5}{6}$, find the common denominator of 30 (6 x 5).

2. Change the unlike fractions to like fractions (Refer to previous page to review changing

unlike fractions to like fractions if you need help.)

3. Subtract the new numerators and place your answer over the common denominator.

   EXAMPLE: 25 - 18 = 7, the numerator. Place 7 over 30. This yields $\frac{7}{30}$.

4. Reduce to lowest terms.

$$\frac{5}{6} - \frac{3}{5} = \frac{25}{30} - \frac{18}{30} = \frac{7}{30}.$$

- ***Subtraction of Mixed Numbers***

Subtract the fractions by changing the mixed number to an improper fraction. For example, to subtract $\frac{3}{6}$ from $2\frac{1}{8}$ you want to change the mixed number ($2\frac{1}{8}$) to an improper fraction.

1. Change the mixed number to an improper fraction. To subtract $\frac{3}{6}$ from $2\frac{1}{8}$ you must change $2\frac{1}{8}$ to $\frac{17}{8}$.
2. Find a common denominator. For the denominators 8 and 6, the common denominator is 48 (6 x 8).
3. Change the *unlike* fractions to *like* fractions.

   $\frac{17}{8}$ becomes $\frac{102}{48}$

   $\frac{3}{6}$ becomes $\frac{24}{48}$

4. Subtract the new numerators and place your answer over the common denominator.

   102 - 24 = 78, the new numerator. $\frac{78}{48} = \frac{13}{8} = 1\frac{5}{8}$.

H. Multiplication of Fractions

Multiplying fractions is easy. All that you have to do is multiply the numerators times each other, and the denominators times each other. For example, if you want to multiply $\frac{3}{4} \times \frac{2}{3}$, you would multiply 3 x 2, to get the new numerator, and 4 x 3, to get the new denominator. This would yield a result of $\frac{6}{12}$.

☞ ***To Multiply Fractions, Multiply the Numerators to Get the New Numerator, and Multiply the Denominators to Get the New Denominator.***

This method of multiplying fractions is sometimes considered to be the "long form" or long method. There is also a "short cut" method for multiplying fractions, called "cancellation." With cancellation, you actually simplify the numbers before you multiply. Look at the example below:

$$\frac{1 \times 8}{4 \times 15}$$

Cancellation can be used because the denominator of the first fraction (4) and the numerator of the second fraction (8) can both be divided by 4. So, if you work the problem, it looks like this:

$$\frac{1 \times 8}{4 \times 15} = \frac{1 \times \overset{2}{\not{8}}}{\underset{1}{\not{4}} \times 15}$$

Once you have canceled all the numbers that you can, you then multiply the new numerators and the new denominators to get your answer.

$$\frac{1 \times 2}{1 \times 15} = \frac{2}{15}$$

• ***Multiplying a Fraction by a Mixed Number***

Whenever you have to multiply a mixed number, you should always convert it to an improper fraction before you work the problem. Remember the rule:

☞ ***When you multiply a Fraction that contains a Mixed Number, change the Mixed Number to an Improper Fraction before you multiply the Expression.***

I. Division of Fractions

Dividing a fraction by another fraction is necessary when you calculate some formulas during college. Follow these steps:

1. Invert the fraction *(flip)* by which you are dividing. This means that $\frac{5}{9}$ becomes $\frac{9}{5}$ below.

$$\frac{4}{5} \div \frac{5}{9} = \frac{4}{5} \times \frac{9}{5}$$

2. Multiply your fractions to get your answer. If you use the example above, your problem now looks like this:

$$\frac{4}{5} \times \frac{9}{5} = \frac{36}{25} = 1\frac{11}{25}$$

3. Reduce your answer to lowest terms and then convert it to a mixed number if it is an improper *(top heavy)* fraction.

• ***Dividing a Fraction by a Mixed Number***

Whenever you have to divide a mixed number, you should always convert the mixed number to an improper fraction before you work your problem.

☞ ***To Divide a Fraction That Involves a Mixed Number, Change the Mixed Number to an Improper Fraction.***

J. Vocabulary Review

Denominator - The bottom part of a fraction. The 6 in the fraction $\frac{2}{6}$.

Numerator - The top part of a fraction. The 2 in the fraction $\frac{2}{6}$.

Simple fraction - a fraction that is not top heavy.

$\frac{2}{3}$ is a simple fraction
$\frac{3}{2}$ is not a simple fraction *(It is an improper fraction)*

Improper fraction - a fraction that is top heavy, such as $\frac{3}{2}$.

Mixed number - a fraction combined with a whole number. Such a fraction looks like the following:

$4\,\frac{2}{3}$. The 4 is a whole number and $\frac{2}{3}$ is a common fraction. Put these together and you have a mixed fraction: $4\,\frac{2}{3}$.

II. Decimals

Medications are frequently prescribed in decimals, and you will find that many of your dosage problems to be solved use the decimal format. A decimal indicates the "tenths" of a number. A decimal's value is determined by its position to the right of a decimal point. In other words:

0.2 is read as 2 tenths because the number 2 is one position to the right of the decimal point.

0.03 is read as 3 hundredths because the number 3 is two positions to the right of the decimal point.

0.004 is read as 4 thousandths because the number 4 is three positions to the right of the decimal point.

The following may help you understand a decimal's position.

Whole numbers	
Ten thousands	10,000
Thousands	1,000
Hundreds	100
Tens	10
Ones	1
Decimal point	.
Tenths	.1
Hundredths	.01
Thousandths	.001
Ten-thousandths	.0001
Decimal numbers	

When reading a decimal, it is important to remember the following rule:

☞ ***Numbers to the Right of the Decimal Point Have a Value Less Than 1 and Numbers to the Left of the Decimal Point Have a Value Greater Than 1.***

To read a decimal fraction, follow these steps:

1. Read the whole numbers to the left of the decimal point.
2. Read the decimal point as "and" or "point."
3. Read the decimal number to the right of the decimal point.

EXAMPLE: 6	.	13	= 6.13
|	|	|	
6	and	13 hundredths	

A. Addition of Decimals

1. Place the decimals to be added in a vertical column with the decimal points directly under one another. If you want to add 0.6, 3.12, and 7, then you would place the numbers like this:

$$\begin{array}{r} 0.60 \\ 3.12 \\ \underline{+\,7.00} \\ 10.72 \end{array}$$

2. Place the decimal in the answer directly under aligned decimal points. Add zeros to balance the columns if necessary. Add the decimals in the same manner as whole numbers are added.

B. Subtraction of Decimals

1. Place the decimals to be subtracted in a vertical column with the decimal points directly under one another. If you want to subtract 4.1 from 6.2, you would place the numbers like this:

$$\begin{array}{r} 6.2 \\ \underline{-\ 4.1} \end{array}$$

2. Subtract the decimals in the same manner as whole numbers are subtracted.

$$\begin{array}{r} 6.2 \\ \underline{-\ 4.1} \\ 2.1 \end{array}$$

3. Place the decimal point in the answer directly under the aligned decimal points. Add zeros to balance the columns as necessary, but not between a number and the decimal.

EXAMPLE: 7.02 - 3.0086

$$\begin{array}{r} 7.0200 \\ \underline{-\ 3.0086} \\ 4.0114 \end{array}$$

C. Multiplication of Decimals

Multiplication of decimals is done using the same method as is used for multiplying whole numbers. The major concern is placement of the decimal point in the answer.

Steps in Multiplying Decimals

1. Place the decimals to be multiplied in the same position as whole numbers would be placed. If you want to multiply 6.3 by 7.6, then place the numbers like this:

```
  6.3
x 7.6
```

2. Multiply the decimal numbers and write down the answer:

```
   6.3
 x 7.6
   378
  441
  4788
```

3. Count off the number of decimal places to the right of the decimal in the two numbers being multiplied and count off the total number of places in the answer. For example:

47.88 two places, count off right to left

This would then read, forty-seven and eighty-eight hundreths.

D. Multiplication by 10, 100, or 1000

Multiplying by 10, 100 or 1000 is a fast and easy way to calculate dosage problems. Simply move the decimal point the same number of places to the right as there are zeros in the multiplier.

EXAMPLES: 0.712 x 10. There is one zero in the multiplier of ten. Move the decimal one place to the right and you get an answer of 7.12.

0.09 x 1000. There are three zeros in the multiplier of 1000. Move the decimal three places to the right for an answer of 90. (Add zeros, if necessary, when moving the decimal to the right beyond the last number.)

E. Division of Decimals

Division of decimals is done using the same method as you use for division of whole numbers. The special concern is movement and placement of the decimal point in the **divisor** (the quantity by which another quantity is divided), **dividend** (a quantity to be divided), and **quotient** (the quantity resulting from division of one quantity by another).

There will be few instances where you will divide decimals to calculate dosage problems. When you divide decimals, the most important thing is placement of the decimal in the quotient. Review this helpful rule.

☞ ***Divide a Decimal by a Whole Number, Place the Decimal Point in the Quotient Directly Above the Decimal Point in the Dividend.***

EXAMPLE: 30.5 ÷ 5

quotient → 6.1
5) 30.5 ← dividend
divisor → (5)
30.
5
5
0

Steps to Divide a Decimal

1. Change the decimal number in the divisor to a whole number. If you want to divide 0.48 by 1.2 you would make 1.2 a whole number, 12, by moving the decimal point 1 place to the right.

   $1.2\,\overline{)\,0.48}$

2. Move the decimal point in the dividend (0.48) the same number of places (1) that you moved the decimal point in the divisor. Divide 4.8 by 12.

   $12.\,\overline{)\,0.48}$

3. Place the decimal point in the quotient directly above the decimal point in the dividend.

   $12.\,\overline{)\,04\dot{.}8}$

4. Divide the equation as if it were a whole number.

   $$\begin{array}{r} .4 \\ 12.\,\overline{)\,04.8} \\ \underline{4.8} \\ 0 \end{array}$$

F. Division by 10, 100, 1000

Dividing by 10, 100, or 1000 is fast and easy. Just move the decimal point the same number of places to the left as there are zeros in the divisor.

EXAMPLE: $0.3 \div 100$.

Move the decimal two places to the left for an answer of 0.003.

G. Changing Fractions to Decimals

Some fractions may divide evenly when converted into decimals. For example, the fraction $\frac{1}{4}$ converts into 0.25 and $\frac{1}{2}$ converts into 0.50. If a numerator does not divide evenly into the denominator, then work the division to three places.

EXAMPLE: With the fraction $\frac{3}{8}$, the 3 (numerator) becomes the dividend and the 8 (denominator) becomes the divisor. Thus,

$$\begin{array}{r} 0.375 \\ 8\,\overline{)3.000} \\ \underline{2.4} \\ .60 \\ \underline{.56} \\ .040 \\ \underline{.040} \\ .000 \end{array}$$

To convert a fraction to a decimal, divide the numerator by the denominator, following these steps:

1. Rewrite the fraction in the division format as shown above; reduce if necessary.

   $\frac{3}{8}$ becomes $8\,\overline{)\,03.00}$

2. Place a decimal point after the whole number in the dividend.

3. Add zeros as needed.

4. Place the decimal point in the quotient directly above the decimal point in the dividend.

5. Divide.

H. Changing Decimals to Common Fractions

When changing decimals to common fractions, the decimal number expressed becomes the numerator of the fractions. For example, $0.75 = \frac{75}{?}$. The decimal number places to the right of the decimal will tell you what the denominator is. For example:

1 place = a denominator of 10
2 places = a denominator of 100
3 places = a denominator of 1000

Therefore, 0.75 is expressed as $\frac{75}{100}$.

To change a decimal to a fraction, follow these steps:

1. The decimal number becomes the numerator.
2. The number of places to the right of the decimal point determines the denominator's value.
3. Write the decimal fraction and reduce if necessary.

EXAMPLE: 0.5 The number 5 becomes the numerator. There is one place to the right of the decimal, which equals a denominator of 10. The fraction becomes 5/10 = 1/2.

I. Rounding Off Decimals

Most decimals are "rounded off" to the hundredth place to ensure accuracy of calculations.

III. Percentage, Ratio and Proportion

The use of percentages is common to many disciplines and frequently encountered in the health care professions.

This section will focus on the basic mathematical skills necessary to calculate percentage problems.

A. Percentage

A percentage:

1. Refers to the number of units of something compared to the whole.
2. Is always a division of 100.
3. Is expressed as the "hundredth part."
4. Is written with the symbol %, which means "of one hundred."
5. Is a fraction where the denominator is 100.
6. Is a decimal by taking the unit to the hundredth part.

The percent symbol can be found with the following:

1. A whole number: 20%
2. A fraction number: $\frac{1}{2}\%$
3. A mixed number: $20\frac{1}{2}\%$
4. A decimal number: 20.5%

B. Fractions and Percents

Sometimes it will be necessary for you to express a percent as a common fraction, or a common fraction as a percent to make dosage calculations easier.

- ***Changing a Percent to a Fraction***

1. Drop the % symbol. 20% to 20
2. Divide the number by 100. $20 \div 100 = \frac{1}{5}$
3. Reduce the fraction to its lowest terms.
4. Change to a mixed number if necessary.

- ***Changing a Fraction to a Percent***

1. Multiply the fraction by 100. For $\frac{1}{2}$, multiply $\frac{1}{2} \times \frac{100}{1} = \frac{100}{2}$.
2. Reduce if necessary. $\frac{100}{2} = \frac{50}{1} = 50$.
3. Change any improper fraction to a mixed number.
4. Add % symbol. 50%

C. Decimals and Percents

Sometimes it will be necessary for you to express a percent as a decimal or a decimal as a percent to make dosage calculation easier.

- ***Changing a Percent to a Decimal***

1. Drop the % symbol. When you drop a % symbol from a whole number, a decimal point takes the place of the symbol. For example, when you drop the % symbol from 68.1%, the decimal point replaces the % symbol.
2. Divide by 100 by moving the decimal point two places to the left. 68.1 = 0.681
3. Add zeros as needed.

• *Changing a Decimal to a Percent*

1. Multiply by 100 by moving the decimal point two places to the right. For 3.19 you would move the decimal point two places to the right, so 3.190 = 319.0
2. Add zeros as needed.
3. Add the % symbol. 319.0 = 319%

D. Ratio and Proportion

A ratio is used to express a relationship between two units or quantities by division. A slash (/) or colon (:) is used to indicate division, and both are read as "is to" or "per." For the ratio 1 is to 2, you can write 1:2 or 1/2. The numerator is always to the left of the colon or slash and the denominator is always to the right of the colon or slash.

A proportion states that two ratios are equal. A proportion can be written as a common fraction form in which the numerator and denominator of one fraction have the same relationship as the numerator and denominator of another fraction. The equal symbol (=) is read as "as." For example:

$\frac{1}{3} = \frac{2}{6}$ 1 is to 3 as 2 is to 6

A proportion can also be written in a colon format in which the ratio to the left of the double colon is equal to the ratio to the right of the double colon. The double colon (::) is read as "as." For example:

1:3 :: 2:6 1 is to 3 as 2 is to 6

To verify that two ratios in a proportion are equal

For a fraction, multiply the numerator of each ratio by its opposite denominator. The sum of the products will be equal.

EXAMPLE: $\frac{1}{3} : \frac{2}{6}$

$$2 \times 3 = 1 \times 6$$
$$6 = 6$$

E. Solving for x

Frequently in dosage calculation problems, it is necessary to find an unknown quantity. In a proportion problem, the unknown quantity is identified as *x*. Read the following word problem and solve for *x*.

Example: Demerol 75 milligrams is prescribed for postoperative pain. The medication is available as 100 milligrams in 1 milliliter. To administer the prescribed dose of 75 milligrams, _____ milliliter(s) would be given.

To Solve for x using a Fraction Format follow these Steps:

1. Write down what is available or what you have in a fraction format. For this example you should write:

$$\frac{100mg}{1\ ml}$$

2. Complete the proportion by writing down what you desire in a fraction format, making sure that the numerators are like units and the denominators are like units:

$$\frac{100 \text{ mg}}{1 \text{ ml}} \qquad \frac{75 \text{ mg}}{x \text{ ml}}$$

3. Cross multiply the numerator of each ratio by its opposite denominator. By doing this, you should get the following proportion:

$$100 \text{ mg } (x \text{ ml}) = 75 \text{ mg } (1 \text{ ml})$$
$$100x = 75$$

4. Solve for x by dividing both sides of the equation by the number before x. In this case, the number before x is 100, so divide both sides of the equation by 100:

$$100x = 75$$
$$x = 3/4 \text{ ml}$$

IV. Algebraic Expressions

Often it is necessary to work with quantities that have a numerical value which is unknown. For example, we may know that Tom's salary is twice as much as Joe's salary. If we let the value of Tom's salary be called t and the value of Joe's salary be j. Then t and j are numbers which are unknown. However, we do know that the value of t must be twice the value of j, or $t = 2j$.

These examples, t and $2j$, are algebraic expressions. An *algebraic expression* may involve letters in addition to numbers and symbols; however, in an algebraic expression, a letter always stands for a number. Therefore, you can multiply, divide, add, subtract and perform other mathematical operations on a letter. Thus, x^2 would mean x times x. Some examples of algebraic expressions are:

$$2x + y, \; y^2 + 9y, \; z\text{-}2ab, \; c + d + 4, \; 2x + 2y(6x\text{-}4y + z).$$

☞ ***When letters or numbers are written together without any sign or symbol between them, multiplication is assumed between the letters and numbers.***

Thus 6xy means 6 times x times y. 6xy is called a term. An algebraic expressions can have several different terms which are separated by + or - signs. The expression 5z + 2 + $4x^2$ has three terms, 5z, 2, and $4x^2$.

Terms are often called *monomials* (mono=one). If an expression has more than one term, it is called a *polynomial*, (poly=many).

The letters in an algebraic expression are called *variables* or *unknowns*.

When a variable is multiplied by a number, the number is called the *coefficient* of the variable. So in the expression $5x^2 + 2yz$, the coefficient of x^2 is 5, and the coefficient of yz is 2.

An *equation* is a condition in arithmetic or algebra where the numbers (1, 2, 3, etc.) or expressions (2x, y + y, etc.) on one side of an equal sign (=) is said to be equal to the numbers or expressions on the other side.

There are four (4) *axioms* (truths) of algebra by which you solve equations.

- **Addition axiom**

If you add the same number or expression to each side of an equation, the equation remains equal.

- **Subtraction axiom**

If you subtract the same number or expression from each side of an equation, the equation remains equal.

• **Multiplication axiom**
If you multiply each side of an equation by the same number or expression, the equation remains equal.

• **Division axiom**
If each side of an equation is divided by the same number or expression, the equation remains equal.

Let's work with these four axioms (truths) to solve some equations. If you master these four axioms, you can solve almost any equation needed in college, and certainly do better on the **NET**.

Some ground rules for solving equations:

1. Dividing or multiplying any number by zero yields a zero. Therefore, this is not helpful in solving equations.

2. Like good parents, what we do to one side of an equation, we must do to the other side of the equation, so that the equation can remain "equal."

3. Our goal is to get all numbers to one side of the equal sign and the letters (representing the "unknown") to the other side of the equation. When we have accomplished this, the equation should be solved.

4. Use the multiplication and/or division axioms to get rid of fractions and get an equation down to one line.

5. Use the addition and subtraction axioms to get the unknown on one side of the equation and the numbers to the other side.

A. Addition Axiom

☞ ***If you add the same number or expression to each side of an equation, the equation remains true or equal.***

A practice problem: x - 15 = 30

Our goal here is to end with the unknown (here represented by an x) on one side of the equation and the numbers on the other side. There are no fractions in this equation, so we turn to the addition and subtraction axioms to remove the number (here a 15) from the left side of the equation containing the unknown.

The equation requests that 15 be subtracted from the x. The opposite operation is addition. Remember that opposite operations cancel each other out, so to speak. We will use the addition axiom and add 15 to each side of the equation. Remember, what you do to one side of the equation, you must do to the other side of the equation. The equation will now look like this:

$$x - 15 + 15 = 30 + 15$$
$$x = 45$$

Check the answer by substituting the value for x (which was determined to be 45 in this case) into the original equation. The equation now balances, and so we have solved the equation, correctly.

$$45 - 15 = 30$$
$$30 = 30$$

Let's solve another equation: $x - 14 = 21$

We want to collect the numbers to one side of the equation and the unknown, the x, to the right of the equal sign. The expression, $x - 14$, implies subtraction; therefore, we use the opposite process, which is the addition axiom. We will add 14 to each side and cancel out the -14.

$$\begin{aligned} x - 14 + 14 &= 21 + 14 \\ x &= 35 \end{aligned}$$

Check the answer by substitution:

$$\begin{aligned} 35 - 14 &= 21 \\ 21 &= 21 \end{aligned}$$

Now you solve the following equations for practice. The solutions are given below.

a. $w - 4 = 8$

b. $m - 12 = 14$

c. $y - 9 = 21$

Solutions:

a.
$$\begin{aligned} w - 4 &= 8 \\ w - 4 + 4 &= 8 + 4 \\ w &= 12 \end{aligned}$$

Check:
$$\begin{aligned} 12 - 4 &= 8 \\ 8 &= 8 \end{aligned}$$

b.
$$\begin{aligned} m - 12 &= 14 \\ m - 12 + 12 &= 14 + 12 \\ m &= 26 \end{aligned}$$

Check:
$$\begin{aligned} 26 - 12 &= 14 \\ 14 &= 14 \end{aligned}$$

c.
$$\begin{aligned} y - 9 &= 21 \\ y - 9 + 9 &= 21 + 9 \\ y &= 30 \end{aligned}$$

Check:
$$\begin{aligned} 30 - 9 &= 21 \\ 21 &= 21 \end{aligned}$$

B. Subtraction Axiom

Our equation for practice: $3 + x = 12$

The equation requests that 3 be added to the x. The opposite operation is subtraction. Remember that opposite operations cancel each other out. We will use the subtraction axiom and subtract 3 from each side of the equation. Remember, what you do to one side of the equation, you must do to the other side of the equation. The equation will now look like this:

$$3 - 3 + x = 12 - 3$$

Then we do the calculation implied (do the subtraction).

3 - 3 (equals 0) + x = 9

$$x = 9$$

Now we have x = 9, which is the answer. Check your answer by substituting the value established for x (which is 9) into the equation and do the calculation.

$$
\begin{aligned}
3 + x &= 12, \quad \text{for} \quad x = 9; \\
3 + 9 &= 12 \\
12 &= 12
\end{aligned}
$$

One side of the equation equals the other side, so we have a true equation and 9 was the value for x.

Let's solve another problem.

$$4 + y = 16$$

Okay. We want to get rid of the 4 on the left side of the equation so that we will have only the unknown on the left side. We will subtract the 4.

$$
\begin{aligned}
4 - 4 + y &= 16 - 4 \\
y &= 12
\end{aligned}
$$

Check the answer by substituting the value for y (which is 12) into the original equation.

$$
\begin{aligned}
4 + 12 &= 16 \\
16 &= 16
\end{aligned}
$$

The equation is balanced, and so 12 is the correct value for y.

Now you solve the following equations for practice. The solutions are given below.

a. $5 + g = 20$

b. $21 + w = 45$

c. $3 + s = 19$

Solutions:

a.
$$\begin{aligned} 5 + g &= 20 \\ 5 - 5 + g &= 20 - 5 \\ g &= 15 \end{aligned}$$
Check:
$$\begin{aligned} 5 + 15 &= 20 \\ 20 &= 20 \end{aligned}$$

b.
$$\begin{aligned} 21 + w &= 45 \\ 21 - 21 + w &= 45 - 21 \\ w &= 24 \end{aligned}$$
Check:
$$\begin{aligned} 21 + 24 &= 45 \\ 45 &= 45 \end{aligned}$$

c.
$$\begin{aligned} 3 + s &= 19 \\ 3 - 3 + s &= 19 - 3 \\ s &= 16 \end{aligned}$$
Check:
$$\begin{aligned} 3 + 16 &= 19 \\ 19 &= 19 \end{aligned}$$

C. Multiplication Axiom

If you multiply each side of the equation by the same number or expression, the equation remains true and equal.

Solve the following equation:

$$\frac{x}{3} = 12$$

A fraction represents the division process. Therefore to leave the x by itself on the left of the equation, use the opposite of division, that is multiplication. Multiply each side of the equation by the denominator.

$$\frac{x}{3} \times \frac{3}{1} = \frac{12}{1} \times \frac{3}{1} \quad or$$

$$\frac{x}{3} \times 3 = 12 \times 3$$
$$x = 36$$

Check this by replacing the variable x with 36:

$$\frac{36}{3} = 12$$
$$12 = 12$$

Let's try some practice problems:

a. $\frac{x}{4} = 5$

b. $\frac{x}{3} = 3$

c. $\frac{x}{2} = 50$

Solutions:

a. $x = 20$
b. $x = 9$
c. $x = 100$

D. Division Axiom

If you divide each side of an equation by the same number or expression, the equation remains equal.

Our problem is $3x = 12$

This equation reads "3 times *x* [an unknown] is equal to 12." This equation then involves multiplication. The opposite of multiplication is division. We will then need to divide both sides of the equation to remove the 3 from the left side of the equation, and thereby leave the letters on one side and the numbers to the other side of the equal sign.

$$3x = 12$$
$$\frac{3x}{3} = \frac{12}{3}$$
$$x = 4$$

Check by replacing the variable *x* with the number 4:

$$3 \times 4 = 12$$
$$12 = 12$$

Let's try another one

$$9x = 27$$

We will divide both sides by 9 to leave the x to the left side of the equation.

$$9x = 27$$
$$\frac{9x}{9} = \frac{27}{9}$$
$$x = 3$$

Solve the following equations for practice. The solutions are on the following page.

a. $5s = 20$

b. $2w = 16$

c. $4y = 28$

Solutions:

a. $5s = 20$

$$\frac{5s}{5} = \frac{20}{5}$$
$$s = 4$$

Check: 5 times 4 = 20
20 = 20

b. $2w = 16$

$$\frac{2w}{2} = \frac{16}{2}$$
$$w = 8$$

Check: 2 times 4 = 8
8 = 8

c. $4y = 28$

$$\frac{4y}{4} = \frac{28}{4}$$
$$y = 7$$

Check: 4 times 7 = 28
28 = 28

E. Negative and Positive Integers

1. Multiplication Rule

- A negative number times a negative number equals a positive number.

$$-3 \times -4 = +12$$

A negative 3 times a negative 4 equals a positive 12.

$$-5 \times -6 = +30$$

A negative 5 times a negative 6 equals a positive 30.

- A positive number times a positive number equals a positive number.

$$+9 \times +11 = +99$$

A positive 9 times a positive 11 equals a positive 99.

+7 x +8 = +56

A positive 7 times a positive 8 equals a positive 56.

• A negative number times a positive number equals a negative number.

-2 x +4 = -8

A negative 2 times a positive 4 equals a negative 8.

+6 x -5 = -30

A positive 6 times a negative 5 equals a negative 30.

2. Division Rule

• A negative number divided by a negative number equals a positive number.

-25 / -5 = +5

A negative 25 divided by a negative 5 equals a positive 5.

-8 / -2 = +4

A negative 8 divided by a negative 2 equals a positive 4.

• A positive number divided by a positive number equals a positive number.

+18 / +9 = +2

A positive 18 divided by a positive 9 equals a positive 2.

+24 / +6 = =+4

A positive 24 divided by a positive 6 equals a positive 4.

• A negative number divided by a positive number equals a negative number.

-14 / +7 = -2

A negative 14 divided by a positive 7 equals a negative 2.

-9 / +9 = -1

A negative 9 divided by a positive 9 equals a negative 1.

- A positive number divided by a negative number equals a negative number.

+24 / -3 = -8

A positive 24 divided by a negative 3 equals a negative 8.

+36 / -9 = -4

A positive 36 divided by a negative 9 equals a negative 4.

3. Addition Rule

- A positive number added to a positive number yields a positive number.

+10 +15 = +25

A positive 10 plus a positive 15 equals a positive 25.

+6 +7 = +13

A positive 6 and a positive 7 equals a positive 13.

- When a positive number is added to a negative number, find the difference of the two numbers and give the sign of the larger.

-10 +6 = -4

A negative 10 and a positive 6 yields a negative 4.

+10 -7 = +3

A positive 10 and a negative 7 yields a positive 3.

4. Subtraction rule

- When you subtract one negative or positive number from another, first, change the sign of the second number, and secondly, follow the rules for addition.

Example:

$$\begin{array}{r} -14 \\ \underline{-\ \ -9} \end{array}$$

To subtract a -9 from a -14, the sign of the bottom number is changed to a positive one. Then the rule for addition says find the difference, which is a 5. Then the sign of the larger number is assigned to the 5, which is a negative sign. The answer is then a -5. The main difference between addition and subtraction of integers is that in subtraction, the bottom number is changed to the opposite one. Then the rules of addition are followed. Simple!

Example:

$$\begin{array}{r} -15 \\ \underline{-\ \ +8} \end{array}$$

The +8 is changed to -8 and the rules of addition are followed. Since both numbers are now negative, the terms are combined and the common sign is given. The answer is -23.

Example:

$$\begin{array}{r} -24 \\ \underline{-\ \ +16} \end{array}$$

The +16 is changed to a -16 and the rules of addition are followed. Since both numbers are now negative, the terms are combined and the common sign is given. The answer is -40.

Example:

$$\begin{array}{r} +22 \\ \underline{-\ \ +12} \end{array}$$

The +12 is changed to a -12 and the rules of addition are followed. Since the two numbers now have different signs, the difference is established as 10. The 10 is given a positive sign because the +22 is larger than the -12. The answer is +10.

Example:

$$\begin{array}{r} -14 \\ \underline{-\ \ -20} \end{array}$$

The -20 is changed to +20 and the rules of addition are then followed. Since the two numbers now have different signs, the difference is established as 6. The 6 is given a positive sign because the +20 was the larger of the two numbers. The answer is +6.

F. Simplifying Algebraic Expressions

It will save time when you are working problems if you can change a complicated expression into a simpler one.

Rules for simplifying expressions which do not contain parentheses:

1. Perform any multiplication or division before performing addition or subtraction. Thus, the expression $6x + \frac{y}{x}$ means add 6 times x to the quotient of y divided by x. Notice that this is not the same as $\frac{6x+y}{x}$.

2. The order in which you multiply numbers and letters in a term does not matter. So 6xy is the same as $6yx$.

3. The order in which you add terms does not matter; i.e.,

   Example: $6x + 2y - x = 6x - x + 2y$
   Example: *4+2=6 as is 2+4=6*

4. If there are roots or powers in any terms, you may be able to simplify the term by using the laws of exponents. For example, $5xy\ (3x^2y) = 15x^3y^2$.

5. Combine like (or similar) terms. Like terms are terms which have exactly the same letters raised to the same powers. So x, -2x, 3x are like terms.

For example, $6x - 2x + x + y$ is equal to $5x + y$. In combining like terms, you simply add or subtract the coefficients of the like terms, and the result is the coefficient of that term in the simplified expression. In the example above, the coefficients of x were +6, -2, and +1; since $6-2+1 = 5$ the coefficient of x in the simplified expression is 5.

G. *Simplifying expressions which have parentheses*

First, perform the operations inside the parentheses. So $\frac{(6x+y)}{x}$ means divide the sum of $6x$ and y by x. Notice that this is different from $6x + \frac{y}{x}$.

The main rule for getting rid of parentheses is the distributive law, which is expressed as $a(b+c)=ab+ac$. In other words, if any monomial is followed by an expression contained in a parentheses, then each term of the expression is multiplied by the monomial.

Example: $2x(y+3) = 2x(y) + 2x(3) = 2xy + 6x$

$x(x-1) = x(x) + x(-1) = x^2 - x$

☞ ***If an expression has more than one set of parentheses, get rid of the inner parentheses first and then work out through the rest of the parentheses.***

Examples:

$$
\begin{aligned}
&2x - (x + 6(x - 3)) + y &&= \\
&2x - (x + 6(x) + 6(-3)) + y &&= \\
&2x - (x + 6x - 18) + y &&= \\
&2x - (7x - 18) + y &&= \\
&2x + (-1)(7x) + (-1)(-18) + y &&= \\
&2x - 7x + 18 + y &&= -5x + y + 18
\end{aligned}
$$

H. Adding and Subtracting Algebraic Expressions

Since algebraic expressions are treated like numbers, they can be added and subtracted.

☞ ***The only algebraic terms which can be combined are like terms.***

Example: $(3x + 4y - xy) + 2(3x - 2y) =$
$3x + 4y - yx + 6x - 4y = 9x - yx$

Example: $(3a + 4) - 2(4a - 3(a + 4)) =$
$(3a + 4) - 2(4a - 3a - 12) =$
$3a + 4 - 8a + 6a + 24 = a + 28$

I. Multiplying Algebraic Expressions

When you multiply two expressions, you multiply each term of the first expression by each term of the second expression.

Example: $(b - 4)(b + a) = b(b + a) - 4(b + a)$
$= b^2 + ab - 4b - 4a$

If you need to multiply more than two expressions, multiply the first two expressions, then multiply the result by the third expression, and so on until you have used each factor. Since algebraic expressions can be multiplied, they can be squared, cubed, or raised to other powers. The order in which you multiply algebraic expressions does not matter.

J. Equations

An equation is a statement that says two algebraic expressions are equal. The following are all examples of equations: $x+2=3$, $4+2=6$, $3x^2+2x-6=0$, $x^2+y^2=z^2$, and

A=2W. We will refer to the algebraic expressions on each side of the *equal* sign as the left side and the right side of the equation. Thus, in the equation $2x + 4 = 6y + x$, the $2x + 4$ is the left side and the $6y + x$ is the right side.

If we assign a specific number to each variable or unknown in an algebraic expression, then the algebraic expression will be equal to a number. This is called evaluating the expression. We can evaluate whether the algebraic equation is truly equal by substituting numbers for the unknowns and then completing whatever addition, subtraction, multiplication or division is indicated. Remember, the correct order for doing these calculations. Maybe this memory trick will help; **M**y **D**ear **A**unt **S**ally - this stands for **M**ultiplication, **D**ivision, **A**ddition and **S**ubtraction. Do your operations in this order.

Order of Calculations

My	=	Multiplication
Dear	=	Division
Aunt	=	Addition
Sally	=	Subtraction

For example,
if you evaluate $2x + 4y + 3$ for $x = -1$ and $y = 2$,
the expression is equal to $2(-1) + 4(2) + 3 = -2 + 8 + 3 = 9$.

If we evaluate each side of an equation and the number obtained is the same for each side of the equation, then the specific values assigned to the unknowns are called a *solution* of the equation. Another way of saying this is that the *choices* for the unknowns *satisfy* the equation.

Consider the equation $2x + 3 = 9$.

If $x = 3$, then the left side of the equation becomes $2(3) + 3 = 6 + 3 = 9$, so both sides equal 9, and $x = 3$ is a solution of $2x + 3 = 9$.

If $x = 4$, then the left side is $2(4) + 3 = 11$. Since 11 is not equal to 9, $x = 4$ is not a solution of $2x+3 = 9$.

K. Review of Equivalence in Algebraic Expressions

One algebraic expression is equivalent to another algebraic expression, if each has exactly the same solution. The basic idea in solving equations is to transform a given equation into an equivalent equation whose solutions are obvious.

Using the four axioms for equations will allow you to solve a linear equation for one unknown in a number of ways. The most common type of equation is the linear equation with only one unknown.

$6z = 4z - 3,$

$3 + a = 2a - 4$

$3b + 2b = b - 4b$

These are all examples of linear equations with only one unknown.

1. Group all the terms which involve the unknown on one side of the equation and all the terms which are purely numerical on the other side of the equation. This is called isolating the unknown.

2. Combine the terms on each side.

3. Divide each side by the coefficient of the unknown.

Example: Solve $6x + 2 = 3$ for x.

1. Using the two rules for solving equations, subtract 2 from each side of the equation. Then $6x + 2 - 2 = 3-2$ or $6x= 3-2$.
2. $6x = 1$.
3. Divide each side by 6. Therefore, $x = \frac{1}{6}$.

You should always check your answer in the original equation.

Since $6(\frac{1}{6})+2 = 1 +2 = 3$, $x=\frac{1}{6}$ is a solution.

If an equation involves fractions, multiply through by a common denominator and then solve. Check your answer to make sure you did not multiply or divide by zero.

Example: Solve $\frac{3}{a} = 9$ for a.

Multiply each side by a, the result is $3=9a$.

$\frac{3}{a} \times \frac{a}{1} = \frac{9}{1} \times \frac{a}{1}$, becomes $3=9a$.

Divide each side by 9,

$\frac{3}{9} = \frac{9a}{9}$, and you obtain $\frac{3}{9} = a$ or $a = \frac{1}{3}$.

Academic Learning Style Section of the NET

The Learning Style Inventory of the **NET** will evaluate which learning style best describes how you learn. While your learning style may be a blend of several approaches, you will, like most students, have very distinctive preferences. You may have a strong visual orientation, or be strongly auditory in your approach to learning. You may be adept at orally expressing yourself, while others may be much more comfortable with written expression. You may be a person for whom "seeing is believing"; if so, you are probably at a learning disadvantage in a setting of oral directions and lectures.

When you are asked to master information in a manner which does not correspond with your personal learning mode, or to study under conditions which interfere with learning, or to demonstrate learning in a manner which does not allow for your individual learning strengths, artificial stress is created, your motivation is reduced, and your performance is depressed.

When the teaching/learning environment attends to your learning style preferences and strengths, your learning will be enhanced. Your achievement may go up, and your frustration may come down.

It is important to identify which learning style works best for you.

The **NET** not only identifies your learning style, but it also identifies the group learning style of your class as you enter school. With the information generated by your diagnostic report from the **NET**, your instructor can compare your individual style against the learning style of the entire class. Thus, the instructor can shape the learning environment that will benefit both you and other members of the class.

A. The Auditory Learner

If you are identified as an auditory learner, you will profit most from hearing the spoken word. You may have noticed that you often vocalize while reading; that is, you move both your lips and throat muscles as you read, particularly when you strive to understand new material. You may feel that if you do not "mouth" the words as you read them, then you are not really reading, and that you will not remember or understand what you have read. Since you best understand and remember words or facts by hearing, lectures for you will be particularly helpful in achieving your academic potential in school.

Learning Hints: If this learning style describes you, then you will benefit from the following approaches to study:

1. *listen to audio tapes*
2. *utilize rote, oral practice*
3. *listen to lectures*
4. *participate in small groups or class discussions*
5. *use a tape recorder to record lectures for further review*
6. *review material, aloud, with other students*
7. *converse with the instructor*

Any interaction activity between you and another person will provide the sound that is so important to your learning style.

B. The Visual Learner

If you understand and remember printed words or facts by seeing them, lectures for you can be particularly difficult. However, if you learn how to take good notes, or are able to borrow class notes from someone who takes good notes, you can effectively learn.

Learning Hints: If this learning style best describes you, then you will benefit from the following approaches to study:

1. *read material in textbooks*
2. *concentrate on the instructor's use of the chalkboard*
3. *utilize teacher, and student, made charts*
4. *watch movies*
5. *use video tapes*
6. *read a variety of books on the subject*
7. *get pamphlets on the topic*
8. *complete worksheets*
9. *study workbooks to identify emphasis on content*
10. *tape record every lecture in order to have an additional opportunity to correct and develop adequate notes*
11. *ask for written course objectives and study the content outline*
12. *develop vocabulary lists so that you can visualize the words and definitions*

If this approach to learning applies to you, write down words and ideas that are given to you, orally, in order to learn by seeing them on paper. Given some time alone with written material, you will probably learn more than in the normal classroom environment.

C. The Social Learner

If you like to study with at least one other person and can not get as much accomplished when studying alone, you would be described as a social learner. Another's opinion and preferences are valued by you. Group interaction for you increases learning and later recognition of facts. Class observation will quickly reveal how important socializing is for you.

Learning Hints: You need to do important learning with someone else. However, the stimulation of the study group may be more important to you at certain times in the learning process than at others.

D. The Solitary Learner

If you like to study alone and actually think best and remember more when you study alone, this learning style describes you. Because you master information alone and form appraisals and make decisions about the information alone, you may often place more value on your own opinions, rather than the ideas of others. An instructor has little trouble keeping you from over-socializing during class.

Learning Hints: If this learning style describes you, then you may benefit from the following approaches to study:

1. *complete important learning, alone*
2. *go to the library or an unused classroom or other such place to study*
3. *avoid group work, as it may cause irritability; group work is distracting*
4. *remember, some great thinkers have been loners*

E. The Orally Dependent Learner

If you speak fluently, comfortably, and seem able to say what you mean, this learning style may describe you. After talking to your instructor about your work, the instructor may find that you know more than paper/pencil tests have shown. You are probably not shy about giving reports or talking to the instructor or classmates; however, writing your thoughts down on paper may be difficult. Organizing and putting thoughts on paper may be a slow and tedious task. As a result, written work (notes from a lecture, reports, themes, care plans, etc.) may appear carelessly done or incomplete.

Learning Hints: If this learning style describes you, then you may benefit from the following approaches to study:

1. *make oral reports instead of written ones, whenever you can*
2. *seek to take oral tests and make oral reports, when possible*
3. *seek to be evaluated by what you can explain, orally, not by written means*
4. *investigate whether you can tape your reports for the instructor*
5. *ask for a minimum of written work, but guarantee good quality*

If your individual test scores are lower than you expected, meet with your instructor and ask to take your next test, orally. You and the instructor may see a real difference in your performance.

F. The Writing Dependent Learner

Do you seek to handle, touch, and work with what is to be learned? Do you feel non-threatened when asked to write essays, and write essay tests, to show what you have learned? Do you feel less comfortable, perhaps even stupid, when asked to give oral answers? Are your thoughts better organized by you on paper than when asked to orally give answers?

If you learn best by experience and a combination of stimuli, this learning style may best describe you. If the manipulation of material, along with sight and sound, makes a big difference as to how you learn, this approach to learning describes you.

Learning Hints: If this learning style describes you, then you may benefit from the following approaches to study:

1. *seek activities that relate to the assignment for re-enforcement*
2. *take careful notes during a lecture, including notes on slides, overheads, pictures, etc.*
3. *involve yourself in physical activities, such as drawing, writing, etc. that require written involvement*
4. *concentrate on perfecting your written reports*
5. *keep notebooks and journals for credit, where possible*
6. *seek to take written tests for evaluation of what you know*
7. *try to have your academic evaluations in a one-to-one conference*
8. *take copious notes during clinical or laboratory instruction*
9. *write out procedures, rather than explain them orally*

Social Interaction Profile Section of the **NET**

This section of the **NET** provides insight into the passive/aggressive, social interaction skills of the entire group of students applying to college. This subtest provides two scores for each student applicant: a Passive and an Aggressive Score. Generally, the *Passive Score* on the **NET** is approximately half the value of the Aggressive Score. This score is not used as part of the entrance criteria for student applicants and is not part of the *Composite Score* generated for each applicant. Instead, a report is generated of the entire entering group of students. This group score can assist instructors to determine whether teaming students for instruction would be helpful in fostering group interaction. This *teaming* of students could prove helpful in teaching students how to work within a group structure striving for success. Remember, the *Composite Score* (Reading and Math) is the score used as part of the admission criteria for new students. You cannot study in order to change your score, and it would not be helpful to your education if you did so. Therefore, simply trust the purpose of this subtest or inventory of the **NET** and answer the questions, openly and truthfully.

Stress Level Profile Section of the NET

This section of the **NET** produces a self-perceived, stress profile for five important areas in personal coping: Family Life, Social Life, Money/Time Commitments, Academic Stress, and Stress in the Workplace. High scores on this profile will indicate areas of personal stress which may cause difficulties for nurses as they progress through college. As a living, functioning human being, you will naturally experience stress. It is helpful for you, however, to occasionally identify those areas which are causing a present and particular stress. The **NET** seeks to help you do this.

Instructors or academic counselors are provided insight into what kind of stressors may be affecting your progress in school if you are performing at a level less than expected, based upon you mastery of reading, math skill and other academic processing skills. An academic councelor could identify with you areas of possible stress and work with you to reduce such stress. This information would also help the instructor when developing problem-solving situations. An instructor could purposely choose a high stress area represented by the whole class, incorporate that stress area into a problem-solving situation, illicit student responses, and work to develop alternatives and options to relieve group stress.

These scores are not part of the entrance criteria for applicants and are not part of the *Composite Score* generated for each applicant.

Remember, the *Composite Score* (made up of your reading and math scores) is the score used as part of the admission criteria for new students. You cannot study in order to change your *Stress Level Profile Score*, and it would not be helpful to your education if you did so. Therefore, simply trust the purpose of this subtest or inventory of the **NET** and answer the questions, openly and truthfully.

Practice Test A
Reading Comprehension

Directions: *Read the following paragraphs and answer the questions that accompany the paragraphs. Circle the letter of the answer which you believe most accurately satisfies the requirements of each question. At the end of this reading test is the answer key.*

A

Grass, the most stepped-on organism on earth, creates more energy than an atomic bomb—just 700 acres of grass gathers from sunlight in one day as much energy as that of the standard atomic bomb or 20,000 tons of TNT. Grass is more valuable than gold and as vital to us as air and sunshine. As a tool against floods, grass is 10,000 times more effective than all the dams built by man.

1. Based on paragraph **A**, which statement is true?

A. Grass is more vital to us than air and sunshine
B. Only an atomic bomb creates more energy than grass
C. A standard atomic bomb is equal to 20,000 tons of TNT
D. Electric power dams are more powerful than grass against flooding

B

Grasses cover one fifth of the land surface of the globe. There are 6,000 species of grass and more individual grass plants than any other kind of vegetation.

2. Which is an inference that can be drawn from paragraph **B**?

A. Grasses cover 25% of the land surface.
B. There are more grass species than any other living thing
C. There are more grass plants than other flowering plants
D. The are 6,000 grass plants, more than any other kind of plant

C

Grasses are simple in structure, consisting of one stem and one leaf on each joint. Few people know that grasses have flowers. Since they are wind-pollinated, their flowers need no color or fragrance to attract insects.

3. Identify the purpose of paragraph **C**.

A. Describe the physical characteristics of grass
B. Reveal that grasses are little understood by most people
C. Reveal that grasses do not need insects in their life cycle
D. Emphasize that grasses need no color or scent to pollinate

D

Grasses are well-equipped for the eternal fight for survival. They are tough, adaptable, productive, quick-spreading, and are found everywhere in polar zones and in deserts, on mountain tops and under water. They produce pollen in huge amounts—up to 50 million pollen grains per plant. Grass pollen, which has been found as high as 4,000 feet in the air, can cover vast distances. It has traveled by air from South America to Louisiana, from Virginia to southern California.

4. Which is a statement of the main idea for paragraph **D**?

A. Grass pollen can cover vast distances
B. Grasses are quick-spreading and are found everywhere
C. Grasses are given what is needed to survive as a species
D. The immense number of pollen grains per plant is the most important survival fact

E

Grass seeds attach themselves to the fur of animals and to the clothes of man. In this way they have followed the trade routes from the Atlantic to the Pacific, from the North to the South. The slave trade brought three grasses, including Bermuda grass, from Africa to the United States because these types were used as bedding for the slaves.

5. An inference that can be drawn from paragraph **E**:

A. The slave trade brought grasses to the United States
B. Bermuda grass came from Africa to the United States
C. Both humans and animals have helped grasses spread
D. Grass seeds followed the trade routes from the Atlantic to the Pacific

F

Grass makes the nutrients of the soil available to livestock, and so to us. In the spring, the grasses draw large quantities of nourishment from the soil, work it over, and store it in their seeds. As the year wears on, the seeds become a storehouse of high-quality food, while the leaves and stems gradually become less nutritious. When the seeds scatter, the better part of the valuable food is lost to livestock.

6. The main idea of paragraph **F**:

A. Humans receive nutrients of the soil through animals
B. Grass makes the nutrients of the soil available to livestock.
C. Grass seeds are the valuable part of a plant for both livestock and humans
D. Seeds become a storehouse of food, and both leaves and stems become poorer eating

7. Based upon paragraphs **B-F**, which is a statement of central theme?

A. Grass seeds carry nutrients from the soil to humans
B. Grasses are well-equipted for the eternal fight for survival
C. Grasses are simple in structure and need no color or fragrance to attract insects.
D. Grasses are prevalent throughout the world, have a tenacity for survival, and are an important source of nutrients for both animals and humans

G

Early in history man realized that grasses offered a way to get high-quality food for himself. All he had to do was to trick the grasses into providing him with the food they store for their own reproduction. When he began cultivating grasses with an eye to eating the seeds himself, the result was the grains from which bread has been made for years. Wheat, corn, oats, rye, and barley are grasses, cultivated from wild and now extinct types. So are rice, bamboo, and sugar cane.

8. The main idea of paragraph **G**:

A. Man cultivated grasses and ate the seeds
B. Grasses offered man a way to get food for himself
C. Man learned to trick the grasses into providing food
D. Wheat, corn, oats, rye, and barley are grasses raised by man

H

These cultivated grasses are the basic foods of man. The Mediterranean culture was based on wheat, the Indo-Chinese on rice, the original American culture on corn.

9. An inference drawn from paragraph **H**:

A. Three basic grasses feed most of the world
B. Northern Europe sought corn as a food group
C. The original American culture ate bread similar to the Chinese
D. Indo-Chinese ate bread from the same grasses as Mediterranean peoples

I

Wheat, the constant companion of Western man for 6,000 years, was introduced into North America by the colonists at Jamestown and Plymouth. Rice, for 4,000 years the staple food of half the world's population, first came to America in 1694 when it was planted in South Carolina. Corn originated on this continent long before Leif Ericson arrived here. It was first given to white settlers at Jamestown. Sugar cane, the greatest vegetable storehouse of energy, was cultivated from a wild saccharine grass in India. It came to the United States from Santo Domingo in 1741.

10. The main purpose of paragraph **I**:

A. Explain the origins of some major grasses
B. Explain how corn came from America to Europe
C. Provide important historical dates in American history
D. Describe how grasses originated in Europe and many other countries

11. The central theme of paragraphs **G-I**:

A. Cultivated grasses are the basic foods of man
B. Wheat has been the constant companion of Western man
C. Grasses are a source of food for mankind throughout the world
D. Early in history, man knew that grasses offered food for himself

J

In manufacturing food, grasses capture energy from the sun and nourishment from the soil. Both are necessary to us.

K

The converted energy of the sun supplies the human machinery with its fuel. When we lift a little finger, drive a car, or build a house, we use energy from the sun which has been stored by plants. We get it by way of meat, milk, or other products from grazing animals.

12. A conclusion drawn from paragraphs **J & K**:

A. Energy from the sun can be converted into usable fuel
B. Manufacturing energy from milk and meat is essential for animals
C. Climbing stairs correlates to both the weight of grass and calories
D. It is important that grasses either capture energy from the sun or nourishment from the soil

L

One pound of pasture grass has enough calories to keep a man walking for an hour and a half, climbing stairs for two minutes, sawing wood for half an hour, or washing dishes for three hours. And the cereal grains provide about four times as much energy as pasture grass.

13. The main idea of paragraph **L**:

A. Cereal grains and pasture grasses provide energy for humans
B. Energy to saw wood for half an hour comes from cereal grains
C. Climbing stairs correlates with sawing wood for half an hour
D. Cereal grains provided four times as much energy as pasture grass

M

Grasses also supply the human machinery with spare parts, in the form of protein. They reach deep into the soil, sometimes as far as 20 feet, to draw out nitrogen and minerals. These they convert into protein—the "stuff of life" contained in all living cells. Protein continuously offsets wear and tear in the body.

14. Which statement reveals the purpose for paragraph **M**?

A. Proteins are the spare parts of the human body
B. Protein is made from nitrogen and other minerals
C. Grasses supply important protein for the human body.
D. Nitrogen can be found by plants as far as 20 feet in the earth

N

Today, the cattle industry in the United States, living off the grass of the land, is a $6 billion business, exceeding in value even the steel and automobile industries. The grazing meat animals, which include sheep and lambs as well as beef and dairy cattle, of the United States produce $12 billion a year in meat and other animal products—seven percent of our gross national production. Conversion of grassland crops into meat produces some 18 billion pounds of dressed beef and veal each year—to the value of over $5 billion. Without grass and hay there would he no milk, butter, cheese, and ice cream, and producing such dairy products puts another $4.5 billion in the pockets of our farmers.

15. The main idea of paragraph **N**:

A. The grazing meat animal industry and its by-products depend on grass
B. Grazing meat animals of the United States produce $12 billion a year in meat and other animal products
C. Without grass and hay there would be no milk, butter, cheese, and ice cream
D. Conversion of grassland crops into meat produces some 18 billion pounds of dressed beef and veal each year

O

Hay production itself "ain't hay" at all— nearly $9 billion worth of this grass crop is produced, annually, which is more than that of any other crop except corn and wheat. Cultivated grass crops—the cereals and sugar cane—add another $9 billion to our income, more than half of it from corn alone.

16. Which statement is supported by paragraph **O**?

A. More hay is produced each year than corn and sugar
B. "Ain't hay" refers to the wealth realized from wheat production
C. A considerable income is realized from the grass crop annually
D. Less than $4.5 billion is realized from the growing of corn annually

P

But the simple, uncultivated grasses, the Jones of the flowering plants, are worth their weight in gold in still other ways. Each year, floods cost the American taxpayer $250 million in damage to crops, equipment, and other property, plus at least another $400 million in lost production. Grass is the cheapest and most effective means of holding rainfall where it hits the ground. In this way it controls floods and, at the same time, protects the soil from being washed or blown away.

17. A point made in paragraph **P** about flood control:

A. Grass is less effective in flood control than dams
B. Grass is the cheapest means of flood control
C. The grass crop in Europe is hurt more each year than in the U.S.
D. More money is lost in damage to crops than in lost production

Q

Grass roots are so fine and extend so far that the roots of a single plant, dug up and placed end to end, would be several miles long. These roots hold the soil crumbs in place with a powerful grip. And they eagerly lap up every drop of water that comes within their reach and keep it in the soil. That's why springs in grassland areas are clear and provide good drinking water—and why dirty water comes from grassless soils, not only unfit for drinking, but carrying off valuable soil as well. Experiments have shown that grassland holds 1,000 times more soil and almost 300 times more water than fields in which a cultivated crop is grown.

18. Which factor in paragraph **Q** supports the topic of soil control?

A. Plant roots hold the soil crumbs in place with a powerful grip
B. Springs in grassland areas are clear and provide good drinking water
C. Grasslands hold 300 times more water than fields of a cultivated crop
D. Grass roots when dug up and placed end to end, would be several miles long.

R

Grasses not only protect land from water and wind. They actually build up land. Cord grasses thrive in the soft mud along the coast, covered by the tide. They break the oncoming waves and catch bits of rocks that are washed in, protecting the shore and building up the floor until it becomes marsh meadow and eventually dry land. Then the cord grasses die out and leave the land ready for cultivation. Much of the tidewater land of Virginia was built that way, and so were the meadowlands on the tidal estuaries in the Gulf of St. Lawrence and Chesapeake and San Francisco Bays.

19. The main idea of paragraph **R**:

A. Cord grasses protect land from water and wind
B. Much of the tidal estuaries in Virginia were built by grasses
C. Cord grasses die out and leave the land ready for cultivation
D. Cord grasses thrive in the soft mud along the coast, covered by the tide

S

Grass, "the handkerchief of the Lord," plays its part in our lives whether we notice it or not. If you are one of the 20 million home owners who sport a lawn, you may curse grass as something that continuously calls for watering and mowing. But if you are one of the 55 million American motorists, you might bless the grass which protects the banks of highways and makes driving safer. If you are one of the two and a half million golfers, you are pleased with grass anyway. But you may not be aware that 750,000 acres of the soft green carpet covers 6,000 golf courses. On baseball and football fields, in parks, picnic grounds, schools, and colleges, grass helps us to relax and enjoy life. We often take our first tottering steps on it, and it closes tightly over our graves.

T

When Edison experimented with his electric bulbs he used a grass—a carbonized bamboo stem—as his first light-providing element, and bamboo fibers were used in lamps as late as 1910. When you tip your Bangkok or Leghorn hat, it is grass which is conveying your greeting. During some periods of fashion the Easter parade saw more grass than hair on ladies' heads, not only in the hats themselves but also in their trimmings.

U

If you buy perfumes, toilet soap, or aromatic oils with the fragrance of violets, chances are that the scent is from the Oriental citronella grass. Grasses are made into mats in China, paper in South Africa, brooms in Mexico, ropes by the American Indians, and thatched roofs everywhere. The uses of bamboo, biggest and strongest of the grasses, include fishing rods, canes and switches, mats, screens, baskets, farm implements, water mains, houses and bridges. Recently bamboo has been used as raw material for cellulose and rayon—the first rayon production from bamboo has started in Travancore, India. It is used in the paper industry in India, Southeast Asia, and France. Due to its fast growth, bamboo pulp yields three times as much paper a year an acre as slash pine.

20. Identify the central, unifying theme of paragraphs **S-U**:

A. Gifts from the grasses
B. The handkerchief of the Lord
C. Use of bamboo used in many ways
D. Edison's experiment with electric bulbs

Rationales for Practice Test A

(Correct responses highlighted in **BOLD.**)

1. A is a poor choice. It states that grass is as vital to us ***as*** air and sunshine, not "more than."
   B is a weak answer because the paragraph states "grass ... creates more energy than an atomic bomb."
   C is the best answer because the paragraph states "... as much energy as a standard atomic bomb or 20,000 tons of TNT."
   D declares just the opposite, that dams are *not* as powerful as grass in restraining floods.

   Type of Question: Inference

2. A is a flawed choice because "one fifth" equals 20%, not 25%.
   B is not a correct inference from the paragraph because grasses were only compared with other plants. No other living species was named.
   C is a valid inference because the paragraph states that "more individual grass plants than another kinds ..." ***Kinds*** **is the key word here and "kinds" could refer to other plants. Based on common logic, the phrase would read, "than other kinds of plants."**
   D is a flawed choice because the paragraph states that there are ***only*** 6,000 species of grass plants, and that there are more *individual* grass plants than all other plants.

   Type of Question: Inference

3. **A is the best answer because the primary information given in the paragraph is the physical characteristics of grass.**
   B lists just one detail among many others presented.
   C is just one detail among many others presented.
   D lists just two details presented among others which were not included in option B.

   Type of Question: Purpose

4. A is only one detail and not a broad enough statement to include the other details listed in the paragraph.
   B is only one detail and is not broad enough to include the other given details.
   C is the best answer because the paragraph develops this concept with supporting details.
   D is only one survival reason of grasses.

   Type of Question: Main Idea

5. A is only a concretely stated detail, not a conclusion or an inference drawn from the paragraph.
   B is a true statement, but it is only a clearly stated detail of the paragraph, not a conclusion or an inference drawn from the paragraph.
   C is the best answer because it includes the two ideas presented for the spreading of grass plants.
   D is a true statement, but is only one concretely stated detail of the paragraph, not a conclusion or inference drawn from the paragraph.

   Type of Question: Inference

6. A is a true statement, but only a detail. The statement lacks emphasis on how plants reap the nutrients of the soil and then pass them on to the animals.
   B is not a good choice for a statement of main idea because the statement neglects to mention the importance of animals passing nutrients of the soil to humans.
   C is the main idea because the details and focus of the entire paragraph develop a theme of the importance of the process by which seeds bring nutrients to both animals and humanity.
   D is a true statement, but not a statement broad enough to include how important it is that nutrients of the soil reach humans through plants or by human consumption of animals who have eaten the plants.

   Type of Question: Main Idea

7. A includes the importance of grass as a source of nutrients for humans, but neglects the importance of grass to animals. Also, B does not include the many other aspects of grass developed in the five paragraphs.
   B includes the topic of grass survival characteristics, but neglects the importance of grass to animals. Also, not included in this answer are the many other aspects of grass developed in the five paragraphs.
   C includes the important topic of plant structure and the part played by color and fragrance in plant reproduction, but neglects the importance of grass to animals and humans as a source of nutrients from the soil. Also, not included in this answer are the many other aspects of grass developed in the five paragraphs.
   D is a statement of central theme because it includes the four facts that support the statement. Therefore, D is the broadest and therefore *best* answer of the ones offered as options.

   Type of Question: Central Theme

8. A neglects to mention that grasses are a source of energy.
   B is the best statement of main idea because it emphasizes that man consumes grasses as a means for gathering energy.
   C is only a fact that grows out of man's discovery that grass can provide energy for him. This is a supporting fact for the statement made as option A.
   D contains examples of grasses, but the statement does not give a reason for man's raising grasses.

   Type of Question: Main Idea

9. **A includes the both the concept of world cultures and that they are fed by three basic grasses.**
   B is not a true statement, based on the paragraph, because the paragraph says that Northern European cultures would have shared wheat, not corn, as a common grass.
   C is not a true statement based on the paragraph which states that the original American culture ate corn, not the rice of the Chinese.
   D is not a true statement based on the paragraph which declares that Indo-Chinese ate rice and the Mediterranean peoples ate wheat.

   Type of Question: Inference

10. **A best summarizes the many details of this paragraph**
    B does not include the other grasses which were given equal importance in the paragraph.
    C is too general a statement and does not focus on the *nature* and significance of the historical dates
    D presents a focus opposite of the one for the paragraph. The paragraph develops the idea of grasses first appearing in America, not that they originated in Europe.

Type of Question: Main Idea

11. A is too limited a focus for central theme. It is just a statement of detail.
B is too limited a focus for central theme. It is just a statement of detail.
C is a summary of the emphasis developed in these paragraphs, which is that grass is an source of food.
D is too limited a focus for central theme. It is just a statement of detail.

Type of Question: Central Theme

12. **A is a true conclusion drawn from both paragraphs, which stress how grasses convert energy from the sun and capture nutrients from the soil. These benefits are then passed on to humans.**
B is not a conclusion because in these paragraphs, milk and meat are only said to be a byproduct from animals, not to be essential for animals.
C is a formula indirectly stated in paragraph L, not J or K.
D is not a good conclusion drawn from these paragraphs because the focus of the paragraphs is not on how important it is for the plants to capture the energy of the sun, but rather how this energy is passed on to meet the needs of humanity.

Type of Question: Predicting Outcomes

13. **A is the main idea of paragraph L because it summarizes an idea supported by the paragraph details.**
B is a true statement but just an idea. It is not broad enough to be a main idea.
C is not the main idea because, although it states a fact, it is only a detail from the paragraph.
D is a true statement, but only a specific detail from the paragraph.

Type of Question: Main Idea

14. A is a true statement, but only a detail of the paragraph.
B is a true statement, but only a detail of the paragraph.
C states the purpose of paragraph M because it states the broad point or purpose developed by the paragraph.
D is a true statement, but only a detail of the paragraph.

Type of Question: Purpose

15. **A is the main idea of paragraph N, as it is a broad statement that develops from the details of the paragraph.**
B is a detail from the paragraph and does not include the other details presented in the paragraph.
C is a true statement, but not one on which the paragraph develops. It does not address the meat byproducts.
D is a true statement, but does not include dairy products and other presented details .

Type of Question: Main Idea

16. A is false. More corn is raised than hay.
    B is false. "Ain't hay" refers to the wealth realized from the production of hay.
    C is true. More than $9 billion as mentioned in the paragraph.
    D is false. More than $4.5 billion is realized.

    Type of Question: Predicting Outcomes

17. A is a false statement. Grass is effective in flood control, but no comparison is made with dams in this paragraph.
    B is true.
    C is a comparison not made or inferred in this paragraph.
    D is false. More money is lost in lack of production than in actual property.

    Type of Question: Inference

18. **A directly supports the topic of soil control.**
    B does not directly support soil control. It just presents the detail about good drinking water.
    C does not clearly support soil control, but, rather, the contrast of grasslands versus cultivated fields.
    D does not directly support soil control, just the length of roots.

    Type of Question: Inference

19. **A is the general idea supported and developed by the paragraph details.**
B is false, based on this paragraph which states that much of the tidal *meadowlands* were created on the tidal estuaries in the Gulf of St. Lawrence, Chesapeake and San Francisco Bays. Much of the tidewater *land* not *estuaries* were built by the grasses in Virginia.
C is a detail, but not broad enough to be the idea around which this paragraph is built.
D is a true statement, but not general enough of an idea to be supported by the other details in the paragraph.

Type of Question: Main Idea

20. **A is the best statement of central theme because each paragraph develops gifts derived from grasses.**
B is just one example of a gift derived from grasses.
C is just one example of a gift derived from grasses.
D is just one example of a gift derived from grasses.

Type of Question: Central Theme

Diagnostic Chart for Practice Test A - Reading Comprehension

Indicate how many questions you answered correctly in each category.

Category	Total Possible	Tally Those Answered Correctly
Main Idea	7	
Inference	6	
Function and Significance		
Central Theme	3	
Purpose of Author	2	
Predicting Outcomes	2	
Total Possible	20	

Multiply 5 times the total questions you have correct. This yields your **final score** for the practice test.

5 x ____ = ____ your final score.

If you earned less than 60 as a final score, study carefully what this study guide teaches about Reading Comprehension, page 9. Re-read the 35 Testtaking Strategies page 18, and then take Practice Test B.

Practice Test B
Reading Comprehension

Directions: *Read the following article and answer the questions that accompany the paragraphs. Circle the letter of the answer which you believe most accurately satisfies the requirements of each question. At the end of this reading test is the answer key.*

A

Equipped with enormous eyes, oversized eardrums and silent wings, he is a superbly engineered nocturnal hunter. He is also one of the most beneficial birds in the air around us. My car broke down in the gloom of a Virginia swamp one night a few years ago. I took out my red warning flashlight and waited for help to arrive. Then, remembering that most night creatures are practically insensitive to red light, I played the flashlight through the deep forest. In the reduced mist I saw a wonderworld of hopping, crawling, running life. Then, suddenly, an instant after my light had flicked past a rabbit, I felt an eerie draft of air—and a great horned owl had seized the unsuspecting animal! I had not heard a sound as the owl went into its power dive. With grim precision, it had captured prey I could not have seen without my light.

1. Which is a statement of main idea for paragraph A?

A. Rabbits are the prey of the owl
B. Most night creatures are practically insensitive to red light
C. A great horned owl can, accurately, power dive in the dark
D. Human eyes can not see in the dark as well as some animals do

B

Owls are rightly known as "lords of the night." Their whole structure is designed around the fact that they must live successfully in the dark, and to this end they have been endowed with some of the most marvelous animal engineering known. With eyesight 100 times as acute as human sight, they can detect an image in the faintest glimmer of light, avoid tree branches and other obstacles and capture the most rapid of darting prey. (At least one kind of owl can capture prey when the light is the equivalent of that thrown by an ordinary candle burning 2,582 feet away!) Their hearing is so acute that they can pinpoint a sound in total darkness. Their powerful claws are set in such a way as to clinch automatically on prey they may not be able to see.

2. The best statement of main idea for paragraph **B**:

A. Owls see in the dark
B. Owls are adapted to survive in the dark
C. The sight of an owl is 100 times as acute as human sight
D. The hearing of an owl is so acute that it can pinpoint a sound in total darkness

C

A wealth of legend has gathered around the owl, and the bird is every bit as amazing as the folklore it has inspired. It is true that owls often inhabit abandoned houses and dark church belfries; for, outrageously hunted by man, they have found refuge there. They have been known to glow with a phosphorescence as they swoop through the gloom; that is because the rotting wood of their nest holes may be coated with luminescent fungi which rub off on their feathers. And the wise old owl is heavy with age; one captive specimen lived for 68 years, a record for birds.

3. Which best state the main idea of paragraph **C**?

A. The owl is heavy with age
B. The owl is an amazing creature
C. Owls do sometimes glow with a phosphorescence
D. Owls often inhabit abandoned houses and dark church belfries

D

Owls are, actually, among the most successful creatures in feathers. Roughly 135 species (18 of them in this country) have colonized all parts of the globe except the frozen Antarctic. Related only distantly to hawks and eagles (their real relatives are the whippoorwills), owls sometimes have wingspans nearly as great as a man's height; sometimes they are as small as sparrows. But we humans, prisoners of the daylight, rarely see owls. And since they do not undertake seasonal migrations, we never see huge congregations of them.

4. Identify an inference that can be derived from paragraph **D.**

A. Owls do not undertake seasonal migrations
B. Owls sometimes have wingspans nearly as great as a man's height
C. Owls are similar in appearance and habits to the whippoorwill
D. Owls can successfully hunt for food on six of the seven continents

E

The screech owl, divided by scientists into 15 races which vary slightly in color and size, is probably the most widespread American owl. Second is probably the barn owl, which has thrived by taking up quarters in human habitations. The largest American owls, the great gray, the great horned and the barred, generally hunt in woods and are rarely seen.

5. Which statement is true based upon paragraph **E**?

A. The barred owl is similar in color and size to the screech owl
B. The great horned owl is seen more rarely than the barred owl
C. Americans see the screech owl more often than the barn owl
D. Americans see the great horned owl more often than the barn owl

6. Which is a true statement based on paragraphs **D & E**?

A. All owls vary slightly from each other in color and size
B. Human prisoners rarely see the great horned and the barred owls
C. Screech owls can have a wingspan nearly as great as a man's height
D. Owls come in a variety of species and are found throughout most of the world

F

During the day, when their specialized gifts are of little value, most owls doze in their roosts or sun themselves on tree branches. Lethargic, they sometimes become open sport for crows and jays, which mob them unmercifully. But so expert is the owl's concealment that he is rarely found.

7. Which is an inference drawn from paragraph **F**?

A. Crows and jays mob owls unmercifully
B. The owl probably does not hunt during the day
C. The owl is rarely found due to its expert concealment
D. "Lethargic" implies that the owl is slow of movement and alertness

G

His subdued coloration resembles sunlight splattering against the bark of a tree, and he can sit so immobile that one ornithologist, after watching an owl for 15 minutes, was convinced that the bird had ceased to breathe. Closer inspection revealed that when the owl inhaled, it compensated for this motion by pressing its feathers more tightly against its body. When it exhaled, it puffed out its feathers. Result: no apparent motion.

8. Identify the main idea of paragraph **G**.

A. The owl is able to disguise its breathing
B. One ornithologist was convinced that an owl had held its breath for 15 minutes
C. Coloration of an owl can resemble sunlight splattering against the bark of a tree
D. The owl presses its feathers more tightly against its body when inhaling and puffs out its feathers when exhaling

9. Which would be a statement of theme for paragraphs F & G?

A. Daytime seclusion
B. Subdued coloration
C. Ornithologists are scientists
D. Open sport for crows and jays

H

For its silent hunting, the owl's body is completely covered with feathers so fine and so soft that they act as mufflers of sound. (Even the base of the owl's immense beak is hidden under a mass of down.) The flight feathers have fuzzy edges, unlike those in other birds, with the result that almost all whir from striking the air is eliminated.

10. The main idea of paragraph **H**:

A. The owl's flight feathers have fuzzy edges
B. The owl's body is covered with fine feathers
C. The owl's feathers muffle the sound of its flight through the air
D. The base of the owl's immense beak is hidden under a mass of down

I

Owls frequently tangle with prey much larger than themselves—cats, porcupines, turkeys. Even the tiny pygmy owl of the Pacific states, a broth of a bird little larger than a bluebird, takes on gophers. How can they do it? Each leg has a thick tendon which runs down it and around a sort of pulley (what in our foot would be the heel), then branches to four needle-sharp talons. When the owl hits its prey, the legs draw up—automatically, from the impact—and the tendon clenches the toes, driving in the talons. The grip is so tenacious that sometimes the only way a person grasped by a stubborn owl can be freed is by cutting the bird's tendons.

11. Which is a statement of main idea for paragraph **I**?

A. The tiny pygmy owl of the Pacific states takes on gophers
B. Each leg of the owl has a thick tendon which runs down it and around a sort of pulley
C. The grip of the owl is so tenacious that sometimes to be freed, the owl's tendons must be cut
D. Owls can hunt prey much larger than themselves because of its ability to clench its toes, driving in its talons

J

Whereas human eyes have both cone cells (which help us to discriminate colors) and rod cells (for light-gathering), the owl's eye is packed tight with rod cells only. These contain a remarkable chemical known as "visual purple," which converts even a glimmer of light into a chemical signal, giving the bird an actual sight impression when a human being would see only the presence of light.

12. An inference that can be drawn from paragraph **J**:

A. Visual purple is a chemical found in the eye of the owl
B. Visual purple converts even a glimmer of light into a chemical signal
C. A sight impression gives more information than detecting the presence of light
D. Human eyes have both cone cells and rod cells. The owl's eye is packed tight with rod cells only

K

The owl's eye is considerably larger than the human eye and does not rotate in its socket. Each eyeball is fixed, like a headlight on a car. So, to see in different directions, the owl is endowed with an extraordinary ability to rotate its whole head.

L

One day I observed a large owl perched on a tree stub in my woods. I suddenly realized that I had made two complete circles of the bird, and yet its head always faced me. An owl can't, of course, swivel its head continuously in one direction. When the neck has revolved as far as it can go—about three quarters of a circle— it whips around to start rotating again. But the action is so rapid that it appears to be one fluid motion.

13. The best statement of main idea for paragraphs **K & L**:

A. The eyeball of the owl is fixed and so the owl rotates its whole head
B. An owl's eye does not rotate, so its head must rotate in complete circles
C. The head of an owl rotates so quickly that it appears to be one fluid motion
D. The owl's eye does not rotate in its socket, but its head does rotate three quarters of a circle

14. Identify the purpose of paragraphs **J - L**.

A. Describe the owl's complex eye parts
B. Explain the owl's extraordinary ability to rotate its whole head to see better
C. Develop the importance of the owl's ability to concentrate completely on its prey
D. Emphasize the visual and muscular skills of the owl that help it survive and prosper

M

For a long time ornithologists could not explain how owls capture prey when there is no light at all. Finally, a graduate student at Cornell University, Roger Payne, proved how they do it. Payne sealed all the openings in a long shed so that it was completely light-tight, spread dried leaves on the floor and then gave a barn owl freedom of the shed. When he turned off the lights and released a live mouse, he heard the mouse move in the dried leaves, then felt a draft of air as the owl left its perch. Immediately he snapped on the lights. The owl had the mouse in its talons.

15. Which is the purpose of paragraph **M**?

A. Describe an experiment conducted at Cornell University
B. Emphasize the importance of the mouse being alive and well
C. Identify who conducted the experiment with owls' night vision
D. Introduce how a graduate student controlled the environment of an experiment with an owl

N

Payne ran experiments to see if the owl was relying on its acute sense of smell, or if it was being helped by invisible heat waves, as rattlesnakes are. All results were negative. Final confirmation that the owl found its prey solely by acute hearing came when Payne plugged one of the bird's ears. Result: The owl went way wide of its mark.

16. Identify an inference that can be drawn from paragraph **N**.

A. All results of the experiments were negative
B. Additional experiments were needed to establish a valid result
C. The owl missed its target when the experiment was conducted in complete darkness
D. An experiment was conducted to determine whether the owl was being helped by invisible heat waves

O

The owl's amazing hearing power comes from the design of its ears. The owl's face is ringed by stiff, curved feathers which collect and bounce sound waves into the eardrums, largest in the avian world. (The ear openings in some species, too, are so large that they entirely cover the sides of the head.) Beyond this, an owl's head is wide, setting the ears far apart, which means that a sound wave will arrive later at one ear than another—an infinitesimal time lapse, but sufficient to give a clue to the direction of a sound.

17. Decide which is a true statement based upon paragraph **O.**

A. The ear openings of owls are so large that they entirely cover the sides of the head
B. Direction of a sound is determined by a sound wave arriving later at one ear than another
C. The owl's amazing hearing power comes from its ring of soft, curved feathers around its face
D. The width of the owl's head is more important for sound detection than the size of the ears or the kind of face feathers

P

To attract their mates, owls must use sound. They have a tremendous variety of calls, and probably no species duplicates another. Their calls are a bedlam of mournful night cries, wails and shrieks. The barred owl can be identified by its maniacal laugh, the great horned by its panther scream, the screech owl by its eerie tremolo. Some of the calls resemble hisses, groans, saw-filing, snores. Burrowing owl young sound exactly like a rattlesnake's buzz.

18. The main idea of paragraph **P** would be which of these four?

A. Owls have a tremendous variety of calls
B. Owls must use sound to attract their mates
C. Probably few species duplicate another's calls
D. Each species can be identified by its night call

Q

An owl in defense of its nest can be a ventriloquist. When Lewis W. Walker, a wildlife photographer, discovered a nest one day, his ears were besieged by sounds of angry bobcats. When that failed to scare him off, the mother would dive from her nest into high grass and make the anguished cry of a small animal in distress. Finally, when nothing else worked, she ripped him with her talons.

19. The best statement of purpose for paragraph **Q** is which?

A. Owls can imitate bobcats and wounded rabbits
B. Introduce a famous wildlife photographer, Lewis W. Walker
C. Owls will imitate different animals to scare off predators from their nests
D. Description of how determined a mother owl can be to protect her nest

R

Studies of owl food habits reveal that owls feed almost exclusively on rodents and other harmful small animals which could overwhelm our crops and forests. Owls are, in fact, among the most beneficial of all birds, rivaling even hawks as controllers of the rodent population. One authority states that in a single night a barn owl may capture as much small prey as a dozen cats. A British study revealed that in one area owls take 23,980 rodents each year per square mile. Nevertheless, only 14 of our 50 states protect all species.

20. Identify a conclusion that can be drawn from paragraph **R**.

A. Owls help to control the rodent population
B. Only 14 of 50 states protect all species of owl
C. Owls can take 23,980 rodents each year per square mile
D. In a single night a barn owl may capture as much small prey as a dozen cats

S

Once common, owls are today being allowed to disappear from the landscape. They are being shot, their habitats are being destroyed by bulldozers and the "landscaping" we now give our woods by removing dead timber decreases their nesting sites. Wouldn't we be well advised to give more respectful protection to these lords of the night?

21. Which is the best statement of main idea for paragraph **S**?

A. Owls need our protection if they are to survive
B. Removing dead timber decreased owl nesting sites
C. Owls are being allowed to disappear from the landscape
D. Owl habitats are being destroyed by road and home builders

Rationales for Practice Test B

(Correct responses highlighted in **BOLD.**)

1. A is a correct inference drawn from the paragraph, but not broad enough to summarize the other details given in the paragraph.
   B is a paragraph detail, but not general enough around which to build the whole paragraph.
   C is only a detail, and does not include a comparison with human eye sight. It is not general enough to summarize the details presented in the paragraph.
   D is a true statement and accurately summarizes the details given in the paragraph.

   Type of Question: Main Idea

2. A is false. The paragraph does not say that owls truly see in the dark. The paragraph explains that they need very little light to see, but they do need at least one candle at 2,582 feet.
   B is a true statement of main idea because the statement summarizes a number of examples of how the owl is adapted to survive during the food gathering process in the near dark or dark environment.
   C is a true statement, but just one example of how an owl is adapted for the dark.
   D is a true statement, but just one example of how an owl is adapted for the dark.

   Type of Question: Main Idea

3. A is a true statement, but only a detail. It is not general enough to be the main or general idea of the paragraph.
   B is a statement general enough to summarize the details of paragraph C.
   C is a true statement, but only a detail. It is not general enough to be the main or general idea of the paragraph.

D is a true statement, but only a detail. It is not general enough to be the main or general idea of the paragraph.

Type of Question: Main Idea

4. A is directly stated in the paragraph, not implied or inferred. Therefore, this statement is not an inference "derived from the paragraph." Concentrate on the direction words of the question, in this case "an inference that can be derived." The question did not ask for a true detail from the paragraph.
   B is directly stated in the paragraph, not implied or inferred. Therefore, this statement is not an inference "derived from the paragraph." Concentrate on the directions words of the question, in this case "an inference that can be derived." The question did not ask for a true detail from the paragraph.
   C is not a true statement because, although the paragraph states that the owl is distantly related to the whippoorwill, it does not suggest any common physical characteristics between the two kinds of birds.
   D is an inference that can a be drawn from paragraph D.

   Type of Question: Inference

5. A is a poor answer choice because the paragraph does not state or imply this at all.
   B is not a true statement because the paragraph says that both are rarely seen by Americans and does not differentiate between the rarity of the two.
   C is true based on the paragraph which states that the screech owl is the most widespread of American owls and lives close to humans. The barn owl takes up quarters in human habitations, both would be widely seen out of the American owl species.
   D is an untrue statement, as the paragraph infers just the opposite.

Type of Question: Inference

6. A is a false statement based on the paragraph and on good testtaking skills, which would suggest that statements containing an absolute, such as *always*, are usually false.
   B is not true. The paragraph states that humans are "prisoners of daylight," not inmates in a correction facility. The paragraph also says that the great horned and the barred owls hunt in the woods and are, therefore, rarely seen.
   C is a false statement based upon the paragraph which states that *some* owls may have such wingspans, but the paragraph does not say which kind of owl has such a great wingspan.
   D is a true statement based on the paragraph which states that there are 135 species of owls and that they are found everywhere in the world except "the frozen Antarctic."

Type of Question: Predicting Outcomes

7. A is practically a word for word statement from the paragraph, not an inference.
   B is not an inference that can be drawn from the paragraph. The paragraph says their specialized gifts are of little value to them during the day, and that they "doze" in their nests. It can be inferred, then, that they are not actively hunting.
   C is not an inference, but clearly stated in the paragraph.
   D is not an inference. The accuracy of this statement depends upon a dictionary understanding of a vocabulary word, not a meaning that can be inferred, accurately, from the context. Therefore answer C is a definition statement, not an "inference drawn from paragraph F."

Type of Question: Inference

8. **A is the best statement of main idea for this paragraph. The entire paragraph develops this idea. This statement summarized the details of the paragraph, and is, therefore, a general statement of the main idea of the paragraph.**
   B is a true statement, but only one detail or example used to develop the main idea of the paragraph. This detail is not general enough to summarize the paragraph.
   C is a simple statement or detail from the paragraph, not the general idea developed by the paragraph.
   D is the opposite of the idea developed by this paragraph. At best, this would be a simple statement of detail, not the general concept around which the entire paragraph was developed.

   Type of Question: Main Idea

9. **A would be a general concept developed by the two paragraphs**.
   B is just one detail given in the two paragraphs.
   C is a conclusion drawn from one paragraph, but does not summarize the general concept tying the two paragraphs together.
   D is just one detail given in the two paragraphs.

   Type of Question: Central Theme

10. A is a statement but does not explain or infer why the feathers are fuzzy.
    B is a true statement, but it does not give a reason for the use of the feathers.
    C is a true statement broad enough to encompass the details that are presented.
    D is just a detail from the paragraph and not broad enough to summarize the focus of the paragraph detail.

Type of Question: Main Idea

11. A is a true statement of detail from the paragraph, but not complete or general enough to summarize the many details of the paragraph.
    B is a true detail from the paragraph, but it does not imply that this is an asset to the hunting ability of the owl.
    C is a true statement based upon the paragraph, but it is just an example of the owl's ability, without stressing this ability as a hunting advantage.
    D is a general statement developed by the details of the paragraph. Therefore, of the available choices, this is the best statement of "main idea."

    Type of Question: Main Idea

12. A is a true detail from the paragraph, but not a conclusion drawn from details. It is simply a restatement of a detail or given fact.
    B is a true detail from the paragraph, but not a conclusion drawn from details, simply a restatement of a detail or given fact.
    C is a true inference from the paragraph. "Presence of light" does not mean an object is detected, only that light, itself, is perceived. "A sight impression" implies that an object is detected. Therefore, the sight impression would give more information.
    D contains true statements and details from the paragraph. However, neither requires the reader to draw a conclusion or make an inference.

    Type of Question: Inference

13. A contains only details from paragraph K and the second clause of this answer is false.

B contains the main idea of the first paragraphs; but, the second statement is not true.
C implies that the head completely rotates, which is not true, based on the paragraph. Also, there is no reference to the main idea of the first paragraph about the eyes not rotating, which causes the owl to rotate his head.
D contains the main ideas of each paragraph, and summarizes the point made in each. Therefore, it is the best statement of main idea for both paragraphs.

Type of Question: Predicting Outcomes

14. A is only one part of the purpose for the three paragraphs. It neglects the discussion of muscular neck motion.
B is just one idea developed in the three paragraphs. It is a very narrow statement of one developed concept, rather than a definition of focus for the three paragraphs.
C is only partially developed in paragraph L, but it is not broad enough to speak to the purpose of all three paragraphs.
D is a general conceptual statement that covers the many details given about the owl's visual and motor abilities.

Type of Question: Purpose

15. A is too vague to be a good statement of purpose. This answer simply states that an experiment was conducted.
B was a factor of the experiment, but the complete darkness, silence, etc., also important, are not included or implied in the statement.
C is too limited to be the general purpose of the paragraph. This statement does not give any reason for the experiment.

D contains information given in the paragraph that, primarily, describes "how" the experiment was conducted.

Type of Question: Purpose

16. A is a stated detail, not an inference.
B is an inference that can be drawn because the paragraph does explain other experiments conducted to achieve a scientific outcome.
C is false. The owl missed its target when one of its ears was plugged.
D is a stated detail, not an inference.

Type of Question: Inference

17. A is false. This statement is written like a absolute. Only some species have such large ear openings, according to the paragraph.
B is a true statement.
C is false. The ring of face feathers is "stiff."
D is a false statement according to the paragraph.

Type of Question: Inference

18. **A best states the main idea. The entire paragraph lists or describes the many different kinds of owl calls.**
B is a given fact, but it does not summarize the many details of the paragraph which list the many kinds of calls.
C is false. The paragraph states: "probably no species duplicates another." Also, the fact is not general enough to summarize all the details and examples given in the paragraph.
D may be a true statement based on the paragraph, but it is not general enough to summarize all the other details given in the paragraph.

Type of Question: Main Idea

19. A contains facts that are only examples supporting a greater purpose.
    B is not the best choice. Walker is identified in the paragraph, but his introduction is too narrow to be the purpose of the paragraph.
    C is a general statement of a purpose achieved by the paragraph.
    D is not the main idea, although it is a valid inference.

    Type of Question: Purpose

20. **A is supported by the facts and examples in the paragraph.**
    B is a true statement, but just a literal restatement of a fact in the paragraph.
    C is a true statement, but just a literal restatement of a fact in the paragraph.
    D is a true statement, but just a literal restatement of a fact in the paragraph.

    Type of Question: Inference

21. **A is a conceptual statement supported by the details of the paragraph.**
    B is a true statement, but the statement is not broad enough to summarize the many facts of the paragraph, which a main idea statement would do.
    C is a true statement, but just one detail. It does not support the plea of needed human protection.
    D is a conclusion or inference that can be made, but the statement is not broad enough to summarize all the facts in the paragraph.

    Type of Question: Main Idea

Diagnostic Chart for Practice Test B Reading Comprehension

Indicate how many questions you answered correctly in each category.

Category	Total Possible	Tally Those Answered Correctly
Main Idea	8	
Inference	7	
Function and Significance		
Central Theme	1	
Purpose of Author	3	
Predicting Outcomes	2	
Total Possible	21	

Multiply 5 times the total questions you have correct. This yields your **final score** for the practice test.

5 x ____ = ____ your final score.

If you earned less than 65 as a final score, study carefully what this study guide teaches about Reading Comprehension, page 9. Re-read the 35 Testtaking Strategies page 18.

Practice Test A
Mathematics

*The **NET** will give you one (1) minute per question to complete this section. Time yourself, but attempt all the problems. The problems begin with basic addition and subtraction of whole numbers and proceed through basic algebra. Work quickly, but carefully. Write your answer directly into this book.*

1. 371
   + 614

   A. 886
   B. 986
   C. 985
   D. 885

2. 4,257
   + 9,368

   A. 13,615
   B. 13,625
   C. 12,615
   D. 12,625

3. 12,817
   + 6,955

   A. 18,772
   B. 18,762
   C. 19,762
   D. 19,772

4. 7,538
   - 2,417

   A. 4,021
   B. 5,021
   C. 4,121
   D. 5,121

5. 735
   - 587

   A. 158
   B. 148
   C. 248
   D. 258

6. 8,015
   - 2,707

   A. 5,308
   B. 5,318
   C. 6,308
   D. 6,318

7. 523
   x 63

   A. 31,949
   B. 32,949
   C. 32,849
   D. 31,849

8. $\begin{array}{r} 623 \\ \underline{\times\ \ 7} \end{array}$

A. 4,241
B. 4,341
C. 4,361
D. 4,261

9. $\begin{array}{r} 703 \\ \underline{\times\ 26} \end{array}$

A. 17,268
B. 17,278
C. 18,278
D. 18,268

10. $6\overline{)936}$

A. 156
B. 156 r3
C. 153
D. 153 r3

11. $7\overline{)507}$

A. 71 r5
B. 68 r5
C. 72
D. 72 r3

12. $56\overline{)14{,}448}$

A. 367
B. 267
C. 358
D. 258

Decimal Operations

13. $\frac{68}{1000}$ as a decimal

A. 6.8
B. 0.068
C. 0.68
D. 0.0068

14. .23 + 1.5 + .002

A. 1.75
B. 1.732
C. 1.352
D. 1.372

15. .17 x .23

A. .0391
B. .391
C. 391
D. 3.91

16. $\frac{.7}{.04}$ is equal to

A. .0175
B. .175
C. 1.75
D. 17.5

17. Hundreth's place in .8951

A. 8
B. 9
C. 5
D. 1

18. $.72 - .57 =$

A. 2.5
B .25
C. .15
D. 1.5

19. Round off to the nearest tenth 3.346

A. 3.35
B. 3.3
C. 3.34
D. 3.4

20.Which is the equivalent decimal number for three hundred ten thousands?

A. 0.031
B. 0.310
C. 3.1
D. 0.0031

Fraction Operations

21. $1\frac{1}{3} + 2 + \frac{3}{4}$

A. $4\frac{1}{12}$
B. $5\frac{1}{12}$
C. $4\frac{2}{3}$
D. $4\frac{1}{6}$

22. $2\frac{1}{6} - 1\frac{1}{8}$

A. $1\frac{1}{24}$
B. $1\frac{1}{12}$
C. $\frac{7}{8}$
D. $\frac{1}{3}$

23. $2\frac{1}{2} \times 3\frac{1}{3} \times 1\frac{1}{5}$

A. $6\frac{1}{6}$
B. $6\frac{1}{30}$
C. $6\frac{1}{5}$
D. 10

24. $\frac{1}{4} \div \frac{3}{2}$

A. $\frac{1}{6}$
B. $\frac{3}{8}$
C. $\frac{2}{3}$
D. $1\frac{1}{8}$

25. Which of the following is correct?

A. $\frac{1}{3} = \frac{2}{5}$
B. $\frac{1}{4} = \frac{9}{12}$
C. $\frac{2}{3} = \frac{8}{12}$
D. $\frac{3}{5} = \frac{15}{40}$

26. Find N for the following: $\frac{N}{3} = \frac{6}{9}$

A. $N = 1$
B. $N = 3$
C. $N = 2$
D. $N = 4$

27. Reduce $\frac{13}{78}$ to lowest terms

A. $\frac{2}{7}$
B. $\frac{1}{6}$
C. $\frac{8}{5}$
D. $\frac{1}{4}$

28. Express $\frac{27}{7}$ as a mixed fraction

A. $3\frac{5}{7}$
B. $3\frac{6}{7}$
C. $4\frac{1}{7}$
D. 4

Percent Operations

29. Two Hundredths as %

A. 20 %
B. .2 %
C. .02 %
D. 2 %

30. 60% of 180

A. 150
B. 388
C. 108
D. 120

31. 7 = (?) % of 28

A. 20
B. 25
C. 75
D. 40

32. 9 is what percent of 27?

A. 25%
B. 40 %
C. 33 %
D. 20 %

33. Two tenths of fifty equals:

A. 10
B. 100
C. 20
D. 25

34. .3% of 60

A. 20
B. 1.8
C. 18
D. .18

35. Ratio of 2 to 5 = (?)%

A. 10
B. 40
C. 4
D. .1

36. $\frac{3}{16}$ = (?)% x $\frac{3}{4}$

A. 20
B. 25
C. 15
D 10

Number System Conversions

37. $\frac{3}{8}$ as a decimal

A. 0.24
B. 0.025
C. 0.375
D. 0.32

38. 0.18 as a percentage

A. 18%
B. 1.8%
C. 0.18%
D. .0018%

39. $\frac{25}{5}$ as a percentage

A. 500%
B. 50%
C. 5%
D. .05%

40. $\frac{4}{5}$ as a percentage

A. 2%
B. .08%
C. 80%
D. 8%

41. $\frac{5.5}{20\%}$

A. 1.1
B. 2.75
C. 27.5
D. .11

42. 0.012 as a percentage

A. 0.12 %
B. 12 %
C. 1.2 %
D. 120 %

43. 12:30 as a percentage

A. 2.5 %
B. 250 %
C. .25 %
D. 40 %

44. $\frac{12}{36}$ as a percentage

A. 33.3 %
B. .333 %
C. 3 %
D. .3 %

Numbers System Conversions

45. 37.5% as a common fraction

A. $\frac{4}{9}$

B. $\frac{5}{18}$

C. $\frac{3}{11}$

D. $\frac{3}{8}$

46. 420% as a decimal

A. .042
B. 42
C. .420
D. 4.2

47. 50 is 20% of x

A. $x = 200$
B. $x = 150$
C. $x = 250$
D. $x = 300$

48. $7\frac{2}{5}$% of x is equal to 74

A. $x = 50$
B. $x = 1000$
C. $x = 100$
D. $x = 500$

49. 25% as a reduced common fraction

A. $\frac{25}{100}$

B. $\frac{4}{16}$

C. $\frac{1}{4}$

D. $\frac{10}{40}$

50. 30% as a decimal

A. 3000
B. .003
C. 3.0
D. 0.3

51. 4 is 25% of x

A. $x = 16$
B. $x = 24$
C. $x = 12$
D. $x = 36$

52. 48% of $x = 60$

A. 175
B. 230
C. 125
D. 120

Algebraic Equations

53. $6a + 3a - 4a$

A. 13a
B. -5a
C. 5a
D. 9a

54. $(x^2 + 3x)-(x^2 + 2x + 3)$

A. $x - 3$
B. $2x^2 + 5x + 3$
C. $5x + 3$
D. $x + 3$

55. $2y + 5 = 27$

A. $y = 12$
B. $y = 11$
C. $y = 16$
D. $y = 8$

56. $2(x + 1) = 3x - 1$

A. $5x = 3$
B. $x = 8$
C. $x = 2$
D. $x = 3$

57. $6bx^2 - 3bx^2$

A. $3bx^2$
B. $- 3bx^2$
C. $9bx^2$
D. $- 9bx^2$

58. $6(t + 3) + 8 - 5(t + 2)$

A. $2t + 36$
B. $t + 16$
C. $t + 36$
D. $t + 13$

59. $3x - 4 = 8$

A. $x = 2$
B. $x = 3$
C. $x = 4$
D. $x = 5$

60. $5m + 8 = 3(m + 4)$

A. $m = -2$
B. $m = 4$
C. $m = 3$
D. $m = 2$

Rationales and Answers for Practice Test A - Mathematics

Circle the problem number in this answer key when you have incorrectly solved a math problem.

*The order of math problems in this test is by skill difficulty, just as they are on the **NET**. Therefore, problem #1 is more basic to your success with math than problem #60. However, mastery of all these skills is very important if you are to manipulate formulas in college.*

Go back to the problems that you missed and try to analyze where your solutions became incorrect.

Next, turn to Practice Test B and complete that practice test.

Question Number	Correct Answer	Skill Evaluated
1	C	Carrying through zero in addition of whole numbers.
2	B	Carrying in addition of whole numbers.
3	D	Basic number facts in addition of whole numbers.
4	D	Basic number facts in subtraction of whole numbers.
5	B	Borrowing in subtraction of whole numbers.
6	A	Borrowing through zero in whole numbers.
7	B	Basic multiplication facts in double digit multiplication of whole numbers.

8	C	Basic multiplication facts in single digit multiplication of whole numbers.
9	C	Multiplication of whole numbers involving carrying through zero.
10	A	Basic short division operations with whole numbers.
11	D	Short division of whole numbers involving zeros.
12	D	Long division of whole numbers.
13	B	Translating a common fraction into a decimal.
14	B	Placing the decimal point in addition.
15	A	Placing the decimal point in multiplication.
16	D	Placing the decimal point in division.
17	B	"Place value" of digits in decimals.
18	C	Placing the decimal point in subtracting.
19	B	Placing the decimal point when multiplying whole numbers by decimals.
20	B	Placing a decimal point in the division of a decimal by a whole number.
21	A	Addition of common fractions and mixed fractions and whole numbers.
22	A	Subtraction of mixed fractions.
23	D	Multiplication of common fractions and mixed fractions and whole numbers.
24	A	Division of common fractions by common fractions.
25	C	Finding equality of fractions.
26	C	Solving for an unknown when dealing with fractions.
27	B	Reduction of fractions.

28	B	Converting a common fraction to a mixed fraction.
29	D	Translating a word phrase into a percentage.
30	C	Calculating the percentage of a whole number.
31	B	Finding what percentage of one number and another number is.
32	C	Finding what percent of one number and another number is.
33	A	Determining the percentage of a whole number.
34	D	Determining the fractional percentage of a number.
35	B	Determining the percentage of a ratio statement.
36	B	Finding what is the percentage of a fractional number and another fractional number.
37	C	Converting a common fraction to a decimal fraction.
38	A	Converting a decimal fraction to a percentage.
39	A	Converting a common fraction to a percentage.
40	C	Converting a common fraction to a percentage.
41	C	Dividing a decimal fraction by a percentage.
42	C	Converting decimal fractions to percentages.
43	D	Converting a ratio to a percentage.
44	A	Converting a common fraction to a percentage.
45	D	Converting a percentage to a common fraction.
46	D	Converting a percentage to a decimal.

47	C	Finding a number when a percentage of it is known.
48	B	Finding a number when a percentage of it is known.
49	C	Converting a percentage to a common fraction.
50	D	Converting a percentage to a decimal.
51	A	Finding a number when a percentage of it is known.
52	C	Finding a number when a percentage of it is known.
53	C	Collecting similar terms with different signs (algebraic addition).
54	A	Removing parentheses and collecting similar terms (algebraic subtraction).
55	B	Solving for one unknown (involving algebraic addition and subtraction and division axioms).
56	D	Solving for one unknown (involving removal of parenthesis through multiplication and then utilization of algebraic addition and subtraction and division axioms).
57	A	Collecting similar terms having exponents.
58	B	Removal of parentheses through multiplication followed by collecting similar terms.
59	C	Solving for one unknown through subtraction and division axioms.
60	D	Solving for one unknown through parentheses removal and followed by the use of addition and substraction and division axioms.

Practice Test B
Mathematics

*The **NET** will give you one minute per question to complete this section. Time yourself, but attempt all the problems. The problems begin with basic addition and subtraction of whole numbers and proceed through basic algebra. Work quickly, but carefully. Write your answer directly into this book.*

1. 481
   + 316

A. 797
B. 795
C. 897
D. 895

2. 5,654
   + 5,728

A. 11,482
B. 11,382
C. 12,482
D. 12,382

3. 8,721
   + 1,893

A. 10,614
B. 10,624
C. 9,614
D. 9,624

4. 8,674
   - 5,213

A. 3,351
B. 3,451
C. 3,461
D. 3,361

5. 826
   - 458

A. 368
B. 364
C. 388
D. 384

6. 7,081
   - 4,690

A. 2,311
B. 2,411
C. 2,491
D. 2,391

7. 472
   x 26

A. 13,272
B. 12,272
C. 13,372
D. 12,372

8. $\begin{array}{r} 582 \\ \underline{\times \quad 6} \end{array}$

A. 3,582
B. 3,682
C. 3,592
D. 3,492

9. $\begin{array}{r} 507 \\ \underline{\times \; 62} \end{array}$

A. 32,534
B. 31,534
C. 32,434
D. 31,434

10. $6\overline{)810}$

A. 135
B. 136
C. 135 r2
D. 136 r2

11. $5\overline{)605}$

A. 121
B. 221
C. 120
D. 220

12. $26\overline{)1{,}322}$

A. 51
B. 50
C. 50 r22
D. 51 r22

Decimal Operations

13. $\frac{56}{100}$ as a decimal

A. 5.6
B. 0.56
C. 0.056
D. 0.0056

14. .3 + .02 + .76

A. 1.56
B. 1.08
C. .108
D. .156

15. .3 x .12

A. .0036
B. 3.6
C. .36
D. .036

16. $\frac{.4}{.02}$

A. 2
B. 20
C. .02
D. .002

17. Thousandths place in .1245

A. 1
B. 4
C. 2
D. 5

18. 0.67 - 0.123

A. .547
B .447
C. .543
D. .443

19. Round off to the nearest tenth 3.163

A. 3.17
B. 3.1
C. 3.2
D. 3.16

20. Which is the equivalent decimal number for twenty eight hundredths?

A. 2.8
B. .028
C. 2800
D. 0.28

Fraction Operations

21. $3 + \frac{3}{2} + \frac{3}{4}$

A. $5\,\frac{1}{4}$
B. $5\,\frac{3}{4}$
C. $4\,\frac{3}{4}$
D. $6\,\frac{1}{4}$

22. $6\frac{7}{8} - 2\frac{3}{8}$

A. $3\frac{3}{8}$
B. $3\frac{1}{2}$
C. $4\frac{3}{8}$
D. $4\frac{1}{2}$

23. $2\frac{1}{3} \times 5\frac{1}{4}$

A. $12\frac{3}{4}$
B. $10\frac{1}{12}$
C. $12\frac{1}{4}$
D. $10\frac{2}{12}$

24. $\frac{3}{7} \div \frac{8}{5} =$

A. $\frac{1}{36}$
B. $\frac{8}{35}$
C. $\frac{15}{56}$
D. $\frac{9}{56}$

25. Which of the following is correct?

A. $\frac{5}{3} = \frac{15}{6}$
B. $\frac{1}{3} = \frac{4}{12}$
C. $\frac{1}{6} = \frac{2}{9}$
D. $\frac{5}{2} = \frac{15}{3}$

26. Find N for the following: $\frac{N}{3} = \frac{3}{9}$

A. $N = 3$
B. $N = 2$
C. $N = 9$
D. $N = 1$

27. Reduce $\frac{45}{75}$ to lowest terms

A. $\frac{2}{3}$
B. $\frac{3}{5}$
C. $\frac{7}{3}$
D. $\frac{5}{3}$

28. Express $\frac{9}{4}$ as a mixed fraction

A. $3\frac{3}{4}$
B. $2\frac{1}{4}$
C. $2\frac{3}{4}$
D. $3\frac{1}{4}$

Percent Operations

29. Express twenty eight hundredths as a %

A. .028 %
B. 280 %
C. 2.8 %
D. 28 %

30. 25 % of 120

A. 40
B. 175
C. 200
D. 30

31. 5 = (?) % of 50

A. 10
B. 25
C. 20
D. 5

32. 6 is what percent of 24?

A. 20 %
B. 25 %
C. 75 %
D. 80 %

33. One fourth of thirty six is:

A. 9
B. .9
C. 90
D. .09

34. 1.4 % of 28

A. .2
B. 3.92
C. .392
D. 20

35. Ratio of 5 to 25 = (?)%

A. 40
B. 60
C. 80
D. 20

36. $\frac{1}{8}$= (?)% x $\frac{5}{8}$

A. 20
B. 40
C. 25
D 12.5

Number System Conversions

37. $\frac{4}{20}$ as a decimal

A. .2
B. .02
C. .8
D. .08

38. 0.7 as a percentage

A. .007 %
B. .7 %
C. 7 %
D. 70 %

39. $\frac{21}{7}$ as a percentage

A. 30 %
B. 300 %
C. 3 %
D. 0.03 %

40. $\frac{1}{8}$ as a percentage

A. .125%
B. 1.25%
C. 12.5%
D. .0125%

41. $\frac{150}{40\%}$

A. 30
B. 0.6
C. 375
D. .3

42. 2.57 as a percentage

A. 257 %
B. 25.7 %
C. 2.52 %
D. .0257 %

43. 2:25 as a percentage

A. .8 %
B. .125 %
C. 12.5 %
D. 8 %

44. $\frac{2}{3}$ as a percentage

A. 6 %
B. .066 %
C. .66 %
D. 66.6 %

Numbers System Conversions

45. 12% as a reduced common fraction

A. $\frac{6}{25}$
B. $\frac{9}{50}$
C. $\frac{3}{25}$
D. $\frac{6}{16}$

46. 12% as a decimal

A. .12
B. 12
C. 1200
D. .0012

47. 75 is 50% of (?)

A. 300
B. 150
C. 225
D. 37.5

48. $4\frac{1}{4}$ % of (?) = 8.5

A. 80
B. 100
C. 200
D. 50

49. 12.5% as a reduced common fraction

A. $\frac{1}{8}$
B. $\frac{2}{16}$
C. $\frac{12.5}{100}$
D. $\frac{25}{100}$

50. 23% as a decimal

A. 0.023
B. 2.3
C. 23
D. .23

51. 12 is 6% of (?)

A. 2
B. 6
C. 200
D. 120

52. $\frac{2}{3}$% of (?) = 33.3

A. 5000
B. 400
C. 600
D. 1000

Algebraic Equations

53. $-6a + 5a + 2a$

A. a
B. 13a
C. -13a
D. 7a

54. $(x^2 + 3x-2) - (x^2 - 2x - 5)$

A. $5x + 7$
B. $x^2 + 5x$
C. $x - 7$
D. $5x + 3$

55. $2y + 5 = 25$

A. $y = 2$
B. $y = 15$
C. $y = 10$
D. $y = 5$

56. $6(x + 1) = 12(x - 3)$

A. $x = 2$
B. $x = 3$
C. $x = 5$
D. $x = 7$

57. $2ax^2 - 5ax^2$

A. $8ax^2$
B. $- 8ax^2$
C. $- 3ax^2$
D. $3ax^2$

58. $6(r + 1) - 2 + 2(r - 5)$

A. $8r - 6$
B. $8r + 14$
C. $4r - 6$
D. $4r + 14$

59. $2x - 5 = 15$

A. $x = 8$
B. $x = 10$
C. $x = 9$
D. $x = 4$

60. $2(m+1) + 3 = (m-2)5$

A. $m = -2$
B. $m = 3$
C. $m = 2$
D. $m = 5$

Rationales and Answers for Practice Test B - Mathematics

Circle the problem number in this answer key when you have incorrectly solved a math problem.

*The order of math problems in this test is by skill difficulty, just as they are on the **NET**. Therefore, problem #1 is more basic to your success with math than problem #60. However, mastery of all these skills is very important if you are to manipulate formulas in college.*

Go back to the problems that you missed and try to analyze where your solutions became incorrect.

Question Number	Correct Answer	Skill Evaluated
1	A	Carrying through zero in addition of whole numbers.
2	B	Carrying in addition of whole numbers.
3	A	Basic number facts in addition of whole numbers.
4	C	Basic number facts in subtraction of whole numbers.
5	A	Borrowing in subtraction of whole numbers.
6	D	Borrowing through zero in whole numbers.
7	B	Basic multiplication facts in double digit multiplication of whole numbers.
8	D	Basic multiplication facts in single digit multiplication of whole numbers.

9	D	Multiplication of whole numbers involving carrying through zero.
10	A	Basic short division operations with whole numbers.
11	A	Short division of whole numbers involving zeros.
12	C	Long division of whole numbers.
13	B	Translating a common fraction into a decimal.
14	B	Placing the decimal point in addition.
15	D	Placing the decimal point in multiplication.
16	B	Placing the decimal point in division.
17	B	"Place value" of digits in decimals.
18	A	Placing the decimal point in subtracting .
19	C	Placing the decimal point when multiplying whole numbers by decimals.
20	D	Placing a decimal point in the division of a decimal by a whole number.
21	A	Addition of common fractions and mixed fractions and whole numbers.
22	D	Subtraction of mixed fractions.
23	C	Multiplication of common fractions and mixed fractions and whole numbers.
24	C	Division of common fractions by common fractions.
25	B	Finding equality of fractions.
26	D	Solving for an unknown when dealing with fractions.
27	B	Reduction of fractions.
28	B	Converting a common fraction to a mixed fraction.

29	D	Translating a word phrase into a percentage.
30	D	Calculating the percentage of a whole number.
31	A	Finding what percentage of one number and another number is.
32	B	Finding what percent of one number and another number is.
33	A	Determining the percentage of a whole number.
34	C	Determining the fractional percentage of a number.
35	D	Determining the percentage of a ratio statement.
36	A	Finding what is the percentage of a fractional number and another fractional number.
37	A	Converting a common fraction to a decimal fraction.
38	D	Converting a decimal fraction to a percentage.
39	B	Converting a common fraction to a percentage.
40	C	Converting a common fraction to a percentage.
41	C	Dividing a decimal fraction by a percentage.
42	A	Converting decimal fractions to percentages.
43	D	Converting a ratio to a percentage.
44	D	Converting a common fraction to a percentage.
45	C	Converting a percentage to a common fraction.
46	A	Converting a percentage to a decimal.
47	B	Finding a number when a percentage of it is known.

48	C	Finding a number when a percentage of it is known.
49	A	Converting a percentage to a common fraction.
50	D	Converting a percentage to a decimal.
51	C	Finding a number when a percentage of it is known.
52	A	Finding a number when a percentage of it is known.
53	A	Collecting similar terms with different signs (algebraic addition).
54	D	Removing parentheses and collecting similar terms (algebraic subtraction).
55	C	Solving for one unknown (involving algebraic addition & subtraction and division axioms).
56	D	Solving for one unknown (involving removal of parentheses through multiplication and then utilization of algebraic addition and subtraction and division axioms).
57	C	Collecting similar terms having exponents.
58	A	Removal of parenthesis through multiplication followed by collecting similar terms.
59	B	Solving for one unknown through subtraction and division axioms.
60	D	Solving for one unknown through parenthesis removal and followed by the use of addition and subtraction and division axioms.

NOTES

NOTES